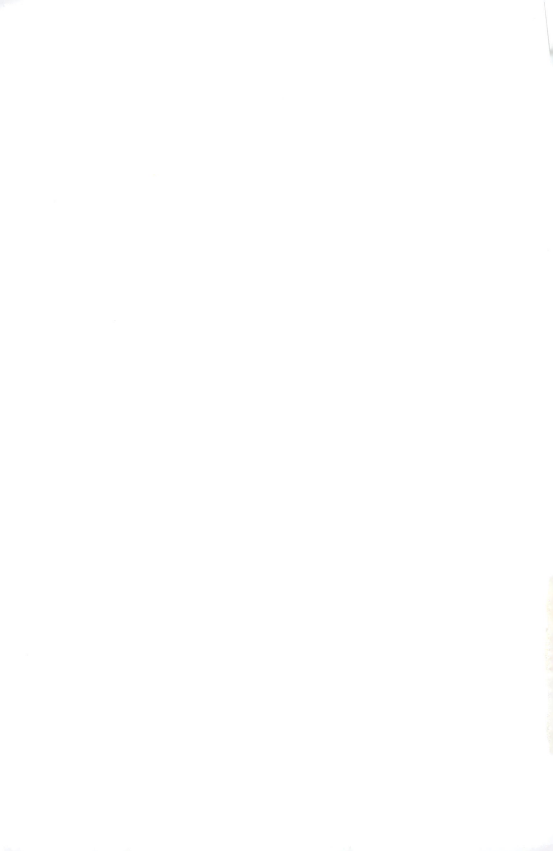

Cancer Causes and Controversies

Cancer Causes and Controversies

Understanding Risk Reduction and Prevention

BERNARD KWABI-ADDO
and
TIA LAURA LINDSTROM

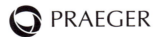 PRAEGER

AN IMPRINT OF ABC-CLIO, LLC
Santa Barbara, California • Denver, Colorado • Oxford, England

Library of Congress Cataloging-in-Publication Data

Kwabi-Addo, Bernard.
  Cancer causes and controversies : understanding risk reduction and prevention / Bernard Kwabi-Addo and Tia Laura Lindstrom.
       p. cm.
  Includes index.
  ISBN 978-0-313-37928-4 (hardback)—ISBN 978-0-313-37929-1 (ebook)
1. Cancer—Risk factors—Popular works.   2. Cancer—Treatment—Popular works.
I. Lindstrom, Tia Laura.   II. Title.
  RC263.K89   2011
  616.99'4071—dc22   2011007870

ISBN: 978-0-313-37928-4
EISBN: 978-0-313-37929-1

15   14   13   12   11   1   2   3   4   5

This book is also available on the World Wide Web as an eBook.
Visit www.abc-clio.com for details.

Praeger
An Imprint of ABC-CLIO, LLC

ABC-CLIO, LLC
130 Cremona Drive, P.O. Box 1911
Santa Barbara, California 93116-1911

This book is printed on acid-free paper ∞

Manufactured in the United States of America

This book is dedicated to the people with cancer who do everything in their power to fight this insidious disease.

—BERNARD KWABI-ADDO

For my dad, Harvey Abell, with love, and in the hope that one day we'll have a cure for cancer.

—TIA LAURA LINDSTROM

Knowledge exists in two forms—lifeless, stored in books—and alive in the consciousness of men. The second form . . . is the essential one.

—ALBERT EINSTEIN

Contents

Preface

Cancer—its name alone can produce dread and hopelessness in those who receive its diagnosis. Yet what we call cancer is really a collection of more than 100 different diseases—each with its own specific origin and prognosis. But all cancers have this point in common: the ability to spread to other locations in the body via the blood or lymph systems. This process is known as *metastasis*. Although a century of intense biomedical research has yielded tremendous breakthroughs, including the discovery of chemopreventive (anticancer) drugs to treat cancer patients, these diseases remain largely incurable.

The scientific community has learned it is contending with a complex and formidable foe. We now know that cancer at the cellular level is a genetic disease, while external and internal conditions that damage DNA can also promote cancer. As the accumulation of several years' DNA damage increases this risk, consequently one of the major risks associated with most types of cancer is age. Another significant factor that influences susceptibility to cancer is a person's genetic inheritance. In some families, a genetic predisposition puts family members at a high risk for particular cancers.

Lifestyle choices can have a tremendous influence on individual cancer risk—in beneficial or detrimental ways. Smokers boost their chances for lung cancer, while those who excessively drink alcohol raise their risk for esophageal cancer. Diet plays a major role in a person's cancer risk. For example, it's thought that diet is in part responsible for the very low rates of prostate cancer among Asian men in their native countries, because second- and third-generation Asian Americans who have adopted the Western diet have a higher incidence of prostate cancer, close or equal to that of Caucasians.

And body fat matters. People who are overweight amplify their risks for colorectal and pancreatic cancers, while those who maintain a healthy, constant body weight and exercise regularly reduce their cancer risks. But in spite of what is known about cancer risk factors, cancer susceptibility can vary greatly on an individual level.

For example, some people smoke all their lives and do not develop lung cancer—while some nonsmokers do. An explanation may be found in the small variations in an individual's DNA sequence known as *single nucleotide polymorphisms* (SNPs). SNPs can affect metabolism positively, such as by enhancing the removal of DNA-damaging toxins in the body, or negatively, by weakening the ability to accomplish such a task. These genetic variants can also influence a person's response to medical treatment. Immune system and stress level, as well as spiritual wellness, can also affect cancer susceptibility.

The good news is that cancer incidence and mortality rates have declined in recent years, mainly due to improved preventive measures. Refrigeration is credited for the drop in stomach cancer, while increasing public awareness about the dangers of smoking is thought to have decreased cases of lung cancer. Declines in colorectal, cervical, prostate, and breast cancer mortality reflect the effect of improved screening, leading to early detection and diagnosis. Thus information about cancer prevention has turned out to be one of the more effective tools to fight this disease and lighten society's cancer burden.

Healthier lifestyle choices such as exercising, eating well, and not smoking or drinking alcohol excessively, as well as avoiding occupational exposure to toxins and infection, are some of the keys to success.

Cancer Causes and Controversies examines some of the risk factors associated with common cancer diseases as well as the current debate over issues such as cancer screening techniques, dietary supplements, and potentially toxic environmental exposures. This book is meant to contribute to the understanding of cancer while increasing awareness of the many measures we may take to prevent this devastating illness.

This book's content is not intended to replace a physician's opinion nor is it meant to guide decision making with regard to screening or lifestyle choices. Rather, it is meant to provide information that may help to avoid various risk factors associated with cancer.

During the research of this book, we were very conscious of the debt we owe to those scientific authors and scholars upon whose work we have drawn. Though we believe that we have been faithful in the spirit of scientific thoroughness, we apologize to the scientific experts for thus simplifying what for many of them represents their life's work. While we have tried our utmost best to use current scientific literature, scientific knowledge is not static—what we believe today may be challenged tomorrow and, at times, proved wrong with the advancement of scientific knowledge.

—Dr. Bernard Kwabi-Addo and Tia Laura Lindstrom

Acknowledgments

To Getty, Ben, Josh, and Dave, thank you for allowing me the much needed time to focus on writing this book. I would like to thank Tia Laura Lindstrom for her help in simplifying the scientific jargon into simple terms for the general public and Debora Carvalko for her insight and suggestions.

—BERNARD KWABI-ADDO

My thanks to Kevin for filling in the gaps, as always. I'd also like to thank my coauthor, Dr. Bernard Kwabi-Addo, for his help in decoding so much medical information. And I'm especially grateful to our editor, Debora Carvalko, for her encouragement and patience.

—TIA LAURA LINDSTROM

Introduction

Cancer's mysteries and miseries have been with us for thousands of years. One of the earliest known references to this collection of diseases appears in ancient Egyptian papyri[1]—medical texts dating from about 1600 B.C. The ancient texts' authors describe swellings and ulcerations that fail to heal, much like cancers we know today.

Little was learned about the nature of cancer during the following 1,500 years. But diagnostic procedures had by the year 1775 advanced enough to enable the English physician Dr. Percival Pott, of St. Bartholomew's Hospital in London, to correlate the development of a specific cancer with prolonged exposure to a workplace toxin. At that time in England, it was common to employ small boys to sweep and clean the insides of chimneys—a treacherous occupation in itself.

In later years, the men who held this job as children experienced a high incidence of scrotal cancer. The doctor discovered that most of his patients with scrotal cancer had worked as chimney sweeps as children and had experienced prolonged exposure to the irritating effects of the soot. This was the first recognized and recorded instance of an occupational cancer due to environmental influences.

But it wasn't until the early 20th century that science began to make great strides in understanding the causes of cancer.[2] This includes the first epidemiological study that linked sunlight to skin cancer in 1907.[2] In 1916 researchers learned that removing the ovaries from a strain of female mice with a high incidence of spontaneous breast cancer decreased the rodents' risk of breast tumors. Later work showed that transplanting ovaries into male mice induced mammary tumors, supporting the theory that hormones in the ovaries could promote breast tumors.

In 1928 scientists identified cervical cancer cells in smears of exfoliated vaginal cells. This discovery led to the development of the Pap smear in 1960, now widely accepted as an effective method of preventing and screening for cervical cancer. Since then, other screening methods for the early detection of various cancers have become routine, such as colonoscopy for colorectal cancer and mammography for breast cancer.

U.S. researcher Dr. Charles B. Huggins made a significant discovery in 1941 when he demonstrated that prostate cancer is hormone dependent. His research showed that physically castrating dogs that had metastatic prostate cancer reduced their disease burden, while injecting male hormones into dogs increased prostate cancer metastasis.

Perhaps the single most important discovery was the identification of deoxyribonucleic acid (DNA) in 1944 as hereditary material. This opened up a whole new realm of science, leading researchers to determine that most carcinogens, agents that cause cancer, do so by damaging DNA or creating DNA mutations.

Since the 1970s, the United States and other parts of the world have taken an aggressive stance against cancer in medical laboratories. This has led to the development of therapeutic treatments such as the antiestrogen drug tamoxifen in 1977. Still used today to treat some types of breast cancer, more than 500,000 people have survived the disease because of this drug. However, the wider use of tamoxifen has been hampered by side effects. In another example, researchers linked prostate cancer with levels of prostate specific antigen (PSA), leading to the creation of the first routine protein biomarker test used in cancer screening and prevention in 1980. Nowadays, several tests screen for the early detection of cancer—a key to successfully treating the disease.

Scientists soon learned that certain bacterial or viral infections could cause cancer. Researchers identified the bacterium *Helicobacter pylori* as a causative agent for stomach ulcer in 1982; it is now known that chronic inflammation caused by this bacterium is a major risk factor for stomach cancer. The human papillomavirus was found to be the causative agent of cervical cancer in 1983. Scientists followed up in 2004 by designing vaccines against the most common tumor-producing (oncogenic) human papillomavirus types, HPV16 and HPV18. It's thought the vaccine could prevent up to 70 percent of cervical cancer cases worldwide.

The completion of the Human Genome Project in 2000 means a great deal to cancer research. As every nucleotide of the human genome has been sequenced and mapped, the way is clear for scientists to learn how cancer cells are different from normal cells. This undoubtedly will lead to understanding individual variations at the DNA level, and it may help explain differences in disease susceptibility. Ultimately, more powerful and specific pharmaceutical drugs could be designed.

Despite this impressive and tremendous progress in cancer research there is still no cure for cancer. This is because cancer is a very complex and sophisticated disease.

As mentioned, cancer is best described as a family of diseases, each with its own locations, beginnings, and progression. These diseases all have a lethal tendency to spread via the bloodstream or lymphatic system to other tissues in a process known as metastasis.

Over 100 types of cancer have been classified.[3] Cancers are usually named for the area of the body where the disease first takes hold, such as in the stomach, lung, or breast. It can be more specific: a cancer found in melanin-forming skin cells and other pigment-making tissues is called melanoma, while cancer in the white blood cells, known as leukocytes, is known as leukemia. Cancers that grow in the body's lymphatic system are referred to as lymphomas.

Approximately 85 percent of cancers are classified as carcinomas. These diseases form in the epithelial tissues—the skin or tissues that line the surfaces of internal organs such as the lung, colon, or liver or ducts in the breast. Other cancers are sarcomas; these arise from cells in bone, cartilage, fat, connective tissues, and muscle.

As their places of origin are diverse, so are the cancers—as well as the major factors that cause these diseases. Skin cancer, for example, can be caused by exposure to the sun's ultraviolet radiation, while breathing tobacco smoke can cause lung cancer. Meanwhile, contact with benzidine, a chemical found in certain dyes, is particularly associated with bladder cancer.

WHAT CAUSES CANCER

Cancer occurs when the normal, necessary process of cell division goes awry because of damage or change in one or more genes of a cell, leading to uncontrolled cellular growth.

In 1928 researchers first proposed that genetic mutation causes cancer;[2] since then great advances have been made in DNA cancer biology. Scientists now recognize that most, if not all, agents that cause cancer (carcinogens) do so by causing mutations in the DNA sequence of normal cells.[4] This is critical, as *healthy DNA is essential for life.* Nearly all known living organisms use DNA as hereditary material, with the exception of some viruses that use ribonucleic acid (RNA).

DNA is a double-stranded, ladderlike helical molecule made up of two chains of nucleotides. Each nucleotide is made up of a sugar, a phosphate, and one of four nitrogenous bases (adenine, guanine, cytosine, or thymine). The arrangement of these bases is the key to genetic inheritance.

All the information needed for normal cell processes, such as growth and division, are contained in these DNA sequences, on genes. Human beings have about

30,000 genes encoded in their DNA. One way that scientists learned that genes play an important role in cancer development is from studying families with members who developed similar cancers through several generations. These families appear to be passing on a gene mutation that carries a high risk of cancer. As researchers have identified several gene mutations that increase a person's chance of developing certain cancers (for example, colon, breast, and ovary), cancers caused by these genes are known as familial cancers. The good news is that only a very small percentage of people in the general population have inherited copies of these abnormal genes, accounting for less than 10 percent of all cancers.

A closer look at how cells replicate may be useful to show how cancer forms at this critical stage. A scientific concept, the central dogma of molecular biology,[5] explains that DNA is transcribed into RNA, which plays an intermediary role in the flow of genetic information from DNA into protein synthesis. Thus, each gene carries the blueprint for constructing a protein molecule. Protein molecules have a role in almost all biological activities in a cell, whether structural or enzymatic. The information flow from a person's genes determines the protein molecule's composition and therefore the functions of the cell being formed.

As all living cells have a limited life span, they must replace themselves through cell division. Cells require genetic information, so DNA must be copied before a cell divides. This process of replication must be accurate as errors could be harmful to the cell. However, mistakes happen. DNA can become damaged. Cells are constantly exposed to harmful agents, some from within the body such as by-products of metabolism or some from environmental carcinogens such as harsh chemicals, tobacco smoke, or UV radiation.

Damaged DNA poses a problem for proliferating cells, whether the injury is from chemical adducts (carcinogens bonded to DNA), double-strand breaks, or a deleted or amplified gene. Cancer cells cannot repair defective DNA. Unrepaired DNA damage can create physical barriers to duplication. When replication does occur, it is likely to be faulty, adding mutations and compounding the problem. This may lead to a loss of genetic information as well as a loss of genomic stability, threatening the survival of daughter cells.

Human bodies have biological safeguards to stop DNA replication of cells harmed by carcinogens so they can be repaired or removed. These are called cell-cycle checkpoints.[6] When these safeguards aren't functioning correctly and the damaged DNA is not repaired, the body risks accumulating new masses of genetically flawed cells. These mutated cells may not respond appropriately to their microenvironment and will likely have a growth advantage over normal cells.

Abnormal cell growth can continue unhindered, forming tumors. Tumors that remain in place and do not spread to nearby tissues are considered benign, not cancerous, while tumors that invade other tissues are considered cancerous (malignant). Benign tumors are not always so; they too can become malignant. Cancer is an efficient colonizer. Malignant tumors can draw oxygen and nutrients to themselves by stimulating the growth of new blood vessels. This process, angiogenesis, is what makes cancer so deadly, as these new capillaries and blood vessels create pathways for cancerous cells to spread to other sites within the body.

Benign tumors can often be tolerated with only mildly debilitative effects; they may also be removed completely through carefully targeted surgery. But metastatic disease poses a more systemic threat by spreading the malignancy to other sites in the body, making complete surgical removal nearly impossible. Typically, cancer becomes lethal when it reaches this stage of uncontrolled growth and diffusion.

Tumors and metastasis are possible because cancer cells can bypass normal biological safeguards—the cell-cycle checkpoints. Cancerous cells ignore signals that normal cells need for growth and survival, and they can avoid immune system surveillance. These lethal characteristics of cancer are collectively known as the hallmarks of cancer.[4]

Certain natural characteristics make some people more likely to develop cancer than others. Inherited mutated genes, a bloodstream with abnormal hormone levels, or a weak immune system are all qualities that acquired even singly may make a person more at risk for cancer.

A mutation in growth-promoting genes, called oncogenes, may instruct cells to divide wildly—much like a car with its gas pedal stuck to the floorboard accelerating uncontrollably. Meanwhile, altered tumor suppressor genes may no longer function properly as brakes for dividing cells and may allow cells with damaged DNA to continue dividing.

Individual susceptibility to environmental carcinogens may also depend on small variations in genes. People differ in their ability to remove carcinogens from their bodies, as well as in their ability to repair DNA damage. These genetic variations can be passed on generation to generation. Higher rates of cancer in some families may also be due to shared conditions such as diet or environmental exposures, including household or workplace carcinogens. For some people, the combination of genetic predisposition and exposure to toxic environmental influences is lethal.

CANCER IS A MULTISTAGE PROCESS

Cancer formation begins when DNA in a cell or population of cells is harmed after exposure to carcinogens. These cancer-producing toxins can come from the person's environment or be a product of regular bodily processes. For example, long-term exposure to viral or bacterial infection may cause chronic inflammation that hurts cells and DNA. Ultraviolet and gamma radiation can also injure DNA. Or a person's normal oxidative metabolism can generate reactive oxygen species (ROS) carcinogens, which in turn can attack DNA.

Many exogenous (from outside the body) carcinogens need to be activated by metabolic enzymes, but detoxification enzymes such as the glutathione

S-transferases also exist to deactivate carcinogens or their intermediate metabolites. People who have inherited genetic variations known as polymorphisms in these types of enzymes may have altered rates of enzyme activation or detoxification, thus increasing or decreasing the carcinogenic potential of environmental exposures. In other words, they will have advantages or disadvantages when it comes to how their bodies deal with carcinogens.

Carcinogens can also induce cancer by affecting epigenetic changes, such as DNA methylation, which alter a gene's activity without changing the underlying DNA sequence.

Once the cancer process has begun, either the cell's defense mechanism detects the abnormality and targets the cell for destruction or the accumulation of further genetic defects helps the flawed cell escape these defenses. The defects may also give these mutated cells a growth advantage, so that they multiply and spread from the site of origin to other sites in the body.

In essence, cancer develops from the build-up of DNA damage and changes over several years and from many causes. This explains why aging is a major risk factor associated with most cancers. Less than 0.1 percent of the total number of cancer cases occurs in people younger than 15, whereas nearly 80 percent of cancer cases are found in people age 60 or older.

Several factors inside the body and in the environment play a role in the development of cancer. Environmental exposure to a variety of natural and manufactured substances makes up at least two-thirds of all cancer cases. These include lifestyle choices such as smoking tobacco, overindulging in alcohol, poor diet, lack of exercise, excessive sunlight exposure, risky sexual behavior, and increased exposure to some viruses.

Other causes may include exposure to certain drugs, hormones, radiation, viruses, bacteria, and environmental chemicals present in the air, water, or workplace. Most chemicals are not carcinogenic, but a wide variety of chemicals can promote the disease.

And so cancer is a multifaceted genetic disease that often requires multiple genetic lesions to breach the body's safeguards. Even people who have inherited flaws in critical protective genes usually do not develop cancer for many years. Yet in many if not most humans the massive accumulation of mutations during a lifetime ensures that some form of malignant disease will eventually develop.

IDENTIFYING RISK FACTORS

Epidemiologists, who study diseases in a population, have been instrumental in identifying risk factors for different cancers. While investigating cancer rates and mortality around the world, they either compare the risk of certain cancers in people with and without particular exposures (cohort studies) or compare the histories of people with and without cancer (case-control studies). This reveals many possible risk factors.

Scientists have learned much through laboratory experiments about how these factors play a role in cancer etiology as well as its progression, often by using animal and human cells in culture or in animal models. One key point researchers discovered is that several significant risk factors for cancer are modifiable for most people. These include a person's work or home environment, sex life, diet (including alcohol consumption), and intake of tobacco smoke.

Add to those factors the pressure exerted on different groups of cells in the body by exposure to viruses, bacteria, and other carcinogens. Cells may also be influenced by hormonal modifications that come from childbirth and birth control. The weight of all these attacks on cellular health can damage normal processes. Yet in principle people have control over most of these risk factors—a few alterations in lifestyle can help prevent many cancers.

This book offers clear information about lifestyle choices that have an impact on the risk for disease. Part I of *Cancer Causes and Controversies* describes the risk factors associated with some of the most frequently diagnosed cancer illnesses, as well as the current understanding of each disease. Part II describes present controversies regarding cancer and nutrition, cancer screening, and dietary supplements and foods for cancer prevention. The text also covers controversies regarding perceived risk factors and cancer—with information that may surprise some readers.

SUMMARY

Cancer creates a tremendous disease burden for the world, claiming millions of people every year around the globe. Yet each time cancer develops, this pervasive disease starts with mutations in one cell. In rare cases, this may be enough to cause cancer, but typically, it takes about four or five mutations to transform a normal cell into a cancerous one.

These mutational alterations can be a single nucleotide change, the deletion of whole genes, or the addition of extra copies of genes, all grouped together to become what's called genomic instability. Particularly for people who have inherited genetic alterations, the buildup of added mutations increases their chances of developing cancer.

A number of mechanisms can leave cells vulnerable to mutations that lead to cancer. Errors can be made when cells copy genetic information during normal cell-cycle activities, or genetic information may be passed unevenly to a cell's two daughter cells. The consequences of these mistakes *can* include the disruption of normal cells' cycle of growth, proliferation, and death.

As a result, cancer cells acquire traits referred to as the "hallmarks of cancer,"[4] or the typical ways cancer cells differ from normal cells. For example, cancer cells do not respond to signals that usually regulate cell growth and division, allowing them to grow unchecked, producing more and more cancer cells. So while cancer cells develop and divide in spite of signals meant to stop proliferation, these mutated cells also learn to grow without the stimulatory signals that normal cells need.

Another hallmark of cancer is how these cells sidestep the natural process of programmed cell death (also known as apoptosis). These cells can also encourage angiogenesis. They can invade other tissue sites by dodging all the checkpoints that confine cells and tissue to their appropriate growth sites. And cancer cells can elude the body's immune system, regardless of the system's constant efforts to locate and eliminate precancerous cells. Although the issue of inherited cancer attracts attention, genetic predisposition to cancer is responsible for less than 10 percent of all cancer cases. Scientists have identified many inherited mutations that may lead to developing particular cancers, such as for breast and colon cancer. Genetics play a significant role in the development of these cancers.

Scientists believe environmental factors are at the root of at least one-third of cancer cases, while one-third to one-half of cancers are considered preventable. This is because many types of cancer are linked to lifestyle choices, such as cigarette smoking. A third of cancer deaths could be prevented if people quit smoking tobacco. After tobacco, being overweight or obese appears to be the next-most-significant preventable cause of cancer. A lifestyle choice linked to prostate cancer is a diet high in red meat, typical of the Western world. Meat cooked at high temperatures can produce DNA-damaging chemicals that may promote cancer development. Liver cancer, meanwhile, is linked to long-term exposure to food contaminants such as aflatoxin, a by-product of molds found on corn and other crops. Cervical cancer can arise out of an HPV infection, especially HPV16 and HPV18, while a major cause of skin cancer is long-term exposure to UV radiation.

Many of these risk factors can be avoided to reduce one's vulnerability to cancer.

In the past 25 years, researchers have made enormous progress in outlining the molecular events that lead to a normal cell becoming cancerous and discovering the critical factors thought to be involved in cancer. Now we know that much of what we put in our mouths and what we do every day affects our risk for cancer.

When people know the risk factors associated with each cancer and take the necessary preventable measures, they can substantially improve their chances for avoiding this devastating disease. And that is the purpose of this book.

Part I

Risk Factors for Commonly Diagnosed Cancer Diseases

Chapter 1

Bladder Cancer

Bladder cancer is one of the first cancers associated with industrial environments. As far back as 1895, German surgeon Dr. Ludwig Rehn noted that people exposed to certain industrial dye chemicals were developing bladder tumors. Later, scientists learned the culprits were carcinogenic aromatic amine compounds called alpha-and beta-naphthylamine (α- and β-naphthylamine) in the dyes.[1,5,8] Bladder cancer continues to have strong links to the workplace today, as will be discussed further in this chapter.

About 70,530 new cases of bladder cancer were diagnosed in the United States in 2010, according to the National Cancer Institute. Nearly 14,700 people died from the disease that year.[9] Those who are at the highest risk for this cancer are male smokers who are older than 65. In fact, the rate of bladder cancer is two to three times higher in men than in women, two or three times higher in smokers than nonsmokers, and like many cancers, the chances of getting this disease increase with age.[1]

Like other illnesses in the cancer family, a large number of cases could be prevented with lifestyle and environmental modifications. This chapter examines these issues in detail, beginning with the biggest and perhaps one of the most modifiable risk factors, smoking tobacco.

SYMPTOMS

People with bladder cancer may find blood in their urine, coloring it slightly or deeply red. People may feel the urge to urinate frequently or more urgently or feel a need to void although nothing appears during attempts.[5]

As the cancer progresses, people may feel abdominal pain as well as aches in their bones. These symptoms are not sure signs of bladder cancer, however, and may indicate infections, benign tumors, and bladder stones as well as other problems.[5] All the same, anyone with these symptoms should see as soon as possible a urologist who can diagnose and treat the disease.

RISK FACTORS

Smoking

Tobacco smoke easily tops all other outside carcinogens when it comes to bladder cancer. Studies show that at least half of those diagnosed with bladder cancer are current or former smokers (although people who quit smoking lower their risk by 30 to 40 percent after one year).[1,3] Childhood exposure to tobacco smoke, even secondhand, also increases risk for this disease, suggesting that children are more vulnerable to the carcinogens in smoke.[3]

Studies indicate that bladder cancers in smokers tend to be larger, be multifocal, and demonstrate higher histological grade and stage. Former smokers retain higher bladder cancer risk than nonsmokers, even 25 years after they've quit the habit.[4]

The more obvious locations for tobacco-related cancer are the lungs or the mouth, and one may well wonder how tobacco smoke can trigger cancer in the bladder. The exact mechanism is not yet understood, but scientists believe the key is how the human body disposes of certain toxins: the kidneys filter the blood and send these poisonous substances out for removal in urine. Essentially, the bladder is like a holding tank for urine, exposing the organ's lining to whatever harmful elements may be stored there. And there could be many. Scientists believe that the body metabolizes more than 60 carcinogenic compounds from tobacco smoke alone, including compounds called nitrosamines (4-amino-biphenyl, acrolein, and oxygen free radicals known to cause tumors in the bladder lining).[1] These often end up in urine, bringing bladder cells' DNA in contact with these carcinogens, which may lead to the genetic damage that predisposes a person to bladder cancer.

Occupational Exposures

Although bladder cancer and industrial workplaces were linked more than 100 years ago (thanks to Dr. Ludwig Rehn, as noted earlier), carcinogenic and otherwise toxic compounds continue to be used today. Aromatic amines are sometimes used in the production of dyes and pigments for textiles, plastics, paints, and hair dyes as well as in drugs and pesticides. Some careers and industries tend to expose workers to more occupational carcinogens: dry cleaners, dental technicians, printers, painters, plumbers, autoworkers, metal workers, textile workers, machinists, and truck drivers and the rubber and leather industries.[1,5,8]

In particular, research has shown that hairstylists and barbers face a higher risk for bladder cancer because of hair dyes and other chemicals used in their work.

Another occupational health threat under study comes in the form of poly-cyclic aromatic hydrocarbons (PAHs), by-products of combustion processes. These occur in a broad range of industries. Some scientists suggest that PAH exposure is responsible for up to 4 percent of bladder cancer cases in European men.[10]

Workers in these occupations face a considerable health risk—particularly men. Some researchers have estimated that up to 10 percent of male bladder can-cer cases in the Western world are due to carcinogens in the workplace. However, a U.S. estimate makes toxic work environments responsible for 20 percent of bladder cancer cases, allowing for latency periods of up to 50 years between ex-posure and symptoms.[1]

Environmental Exposures

Just because something is natural, it doesn't mean it's safe. Arsenic is found throughout the natural environment and can contaminate groundwater supplies. Studies have confirmed that inorganic arsenic (considered more harmful than the organic form) can trigger skin cancer or lung cancer.[1] Research in Taiwan has also pointed to an increased risk of urinary tract cancer from high levels of arsenic in well water.[6]

The use of nitrogen-based fertilizers and pesticides can eventually contaminate well water with nitrates.[1] Some studies from Spain and the United States have shown a correlation between higher nitrate levels in drinking water and a rise in bladder cancer cases, although other studies have not confirmed these results. More research on drinking water and these contaminants is needed.[6]

Parasites

Most bladder cancer cases in the developing world are caused by parasites, par-ticularly *schistosomiasis hematobium,* prevalent in Egypt's Nile River valley and other parts of Africa.[2,5] However, a parasitic infection leading to bladder cancer is rare in the developed world; tobacco smoke or workplace toxins are much more likely causes of this disease.[2]

Cancer Treatments

It is a cruel irony that the treatment for one form of cancer may trigger another. Some therapeutic agents such as cyclophosphamide and arsenic increase the pa-tient's risk for bladder cancer, as do radiotherapy treatments to the pelvic area for the treatment of cervical cancer, prostate cancer, and other cancers of the lower body.[5] It is important to note that a very small proportion of bladder cancer cases are associated with these treatments.

Family or Ethnic Group

Caucasians are twice as likely to get bladder cancer as African Americans or Hispanics, while Asians have the lowest rates of this disease. People with a family history of bladder cancer may have inherited a mutated gene, although this is uncommon. Those with a first-degree relative such as a parent or sibling with bladder cancer appear to have a slightly higher risk of getting this disease—but in many cases it may be high-risk lifestyle habits that have been inherited, not faulty genes.[5]

Genetic Factors

In rare cases risk for bladder cancer can be affected by mutations in genes responsible for DNA repair and the removal of carcinogens. If the repair genes are harmed, they may not be able to correct damaged DNA, and a situation of genomic instability develops. Likewise, a buildup of carcinogens can predispose someone to cancer. These mutations may not necessarily be inherited.

FACTORS THAT MAY LOWER BLADDER CANCER RISK

Eat Vegetables and Fruit, Avoid Saturated Fat

Studies show that eating plenty of fruit and vegetables lowers the chances of getting bladder cancer. Some research suggests that fruit-and-veggie eaters cut their risk of bladder cancer in half. Vegetables appear to have the most protective benefits, especially green and yellow varieties; nonsmokers seem to profit the most from eating this way. Other research has shown that those who eat the highest levels of saturated fats have a markedly higher risk of this cancer type. However, the increased threat from a diet soaked in saturated fats could also be due to the high calorie count.[1]

Drink Water

Some research indicates that drinking more fluids may lessen a person's risk for bladder cancer. As carcinogens in urine are thought to be one of the causes of this disease, one theory is that by diluting the urine and therefore increasing urination, the contact time the bladder has with carcinogens is shortened. This could prevent DNA damage in the bladder tissue. Researchers have suggested six glasses of water per day as the beneficial dosage. Other studies, however, have not demonstrated a significant correlation between increased fluid intake and lower bladder cancer risk. The topic remains controversial.[1,7]

Drink Green Tea

Studies show green tea drinkers have a lower risk of bladder cancer—hence the low rates of this disease in Asia. Scientists note that, after two generations in the United States, families who have emigrated from Japan have a doubled risk of bladder cancer.[1] In the laboratory, researchers with in vitro (in test tube) cell cultures and human subjects have demonstrated how green tea's polyphenols interfere with several processes that can lead to DNA damage and possibly cancer.[1]

SUMMARY

Although the causes of bladder cancer are not yet fully understood, it's well known that some members of the population are more vulnerable to this disease than others. It may be because they are exposed to certain environmental risk factors, such as tobacco smoke or particular chemical agents. Therefore, you can reduce exposure to carcinogens and lessen risk for this disease by quitting smoking, avoiding secondhand smoke, and avoiding or altering a toxic work environment.

Still, most people with known risk factors do not get bladder cancer. And many who do get this disease have no risk factors.

Chapter 2

Brain Cancer

While only about 2 percent of adult cancer patients have brain cancer, this disease has a devastating impact: it's the second-most-common cancer in children under age 15—amounting to 20 percent of childhood cancers.[1]

Brain cancer is named for cancer that begins in the brain or the central spinal canal. Cancers that begin elsewhere in the body and then spread to the brain are called metastatic brain tumors. Not all brain tumors are cancerous or malignant, but they can become so. Even benign brain tumors may be a problem because they are growing within a limited and contained space, the skull. The focus of this chapter, however, is on malignant brain tumors.

Brain cancer is an umbrella term for more than 120 different central nervous system (CNS) tumors of the brain and spinal cord, according to data from the National Brain Tumor Society.[13] These tumors do not necessarily form inside the brain but on tissues essential to brain function, such as tissues covering the paraspinal nerves (tumors called schwannomas) or tissues covering membranes (tumors called meningiomas). Primary brain tumors—those originating in the brain—can take the form of a benign meningioma in the tissue covering the brain (the dura) or a glioma (or glioblastoma, the most common and aggressive brain cancer), which first grows in the glia cells that surround the neurons throughout the brain.

SYMPTOMS

Brain tumor symptoms depend on the kind of tumor the person has, where it is located, and its size. Generally, people with brain tumors experience headaches, nausea, and vomiting. They may have problems with memory, hearing, vision, speech, balance, walking, or concentrating and may experience muscle twitching (or seizures) and changes in mood and personality. These are known as neurocognitive symptoms as they are generated by problems on the neuropathway. A person with a brain tumor may also feel numbness or tingling in limbs. It's important to note that symptoms such as these could be caused by problems other than brain tumors.

TREATMENT CHALLENGES

Unfortunately, brain cancer is difficult to treat. As it concerns the human body's most vital organ—the seat of the five senses, emotion, thought, and movement—using surgery to remove all or part of diseased tissue can damage essential brain functions. This difficulty is compounded by the way cancer spreads into various key areas of the brain. As the brain is located within a hard, bony enclosure (the skull), tumors do not have much room to grow without putting pressure on blood vessels or healthy brain tissue, further complicating medical efforts. Another problem is that most brain cancers do not respond to chemotherapy or radiation, treatments often used successfully with other cancers.

RISK FACTORS

Ethnic Group

Brain cancer is more common in the developed world than in developing countries, and Caucasians, particularly males, have the highest incidence and mortality rates for this disease.[1] In general, men in all ethnic groups are at greater risk for brain cancer than women, although women are more at risk for meningiomas. On average, men and women are diagnosed with primary brain tumors at age 54, although the onset of a glioma or meningioma typically begins at age 62.

Gender and Hormonal Factors

Hormonal factors may influence brain cancer risk, particularly for men. Three-quarters of adult primary brain tumors are gliomas—a tumor type occurring one and a half times more often in males, according to several studies.[16] Why men are at a higher risk for brain cancer remains to be understood. The results of one study suggest that reproductive hormones may be involved in the development of glioma in women.[5] Researchers found that postmenopausal women have an increased risk for this cancer, especially if they started menstruation at a later age. Women who used hormone therapy to treat menopausal symptoms have a decreased risk of glioma compared to women who didn't use hormones. The study also found that women who had breast-fed their children for more than 18 months total in their lives increased their risk for glioma, compared to women who had never breast-fed.[16]

Other studies also show a lower risk of glioma in the female population compared to the male population. These studies suggest gender's protective effect on women begins around the onset of menstruation, becomes strongest near meno-pause, and then decreases in the postmenopausal years.[6]

The gender difference regarding cancer risk crosses ethnic groups and there-fore discounts the idea that environmental factors could play a role. This raises the question of whether female hormones help prevent brain cancer or whether male hormones help promote the cancer. Genetic differences may also influence brain cancer development in men and women.

GENETIC AND HEREDITARY RISK FACTORS

Research suggests that some people may be genetically predisposed to brain cancer, although this accounts for less than 10 percent of cases.

Those who have a family history of brain cancer seem to have a higher risk, es-pecially when parents or siblings (first-degree relatives) have the disease. Reports of this link are inconsistent, however. More evidence supports the link between brain cancer and several rare diseases that are passed down through families. These include neurofibromatosis types 1 (NF1) and 2 (NF2), tuberous sclerosis complex, von Hippel–Lindau disease and the even less common Cowden disease, and Li-Fraumeni and Gorlin syndromes.[2,8]

For the sake of simplicity, the most common of these rare syndromes, NF1 and NF2 and Li-Fraumeni syndrome, are discussed here.

Neurofibromatosis Types 1 and 2

An inherited disease, neurofibromatosis causes nerve cells (Schwann cells) to grow tumors called neurofibromas that may be destructive if they press on nerves or other tissues. A person with this disease may develop bumps under the skin, colored areas (such as café au lait marks), spinal or skeletal problems, or other neurological issues. Distinct for its particular skin characteristics, type 1 (NF1) is the most common type, occurring in about 1 in 4,000 people.

Type 2 (NF2) has a less obvious appearance on the skin; its characteristics include bilateral acoustic neuromas (benign tumors of the acoustic, or hearing, nerve) and spinal gliomas. This form of neurofibromatosis is much less common than type 1 and found in about 1 in 40,000 people.

Li-Fraumeni Cancer Syndrome

Li-Fraumeni cancer syndrome is a heritable disease typically caused by a mu-tation in a key gene, *p53*, a tumor suppressor gene that is also involved in DNA repair. Although it contributes minimally to brain tumor cases, this syndrome has been connected with primary cancers such as sarcoma, breast cancer, leukemia, and brain cancer.

In spite of the hereditary connection between these diseases and brain cancer, not all people with these genetic predispositions will develop brain cancer.

Familial Diseases and Genetic Mutations

Some of the genetic mutations linked to these rare, inherited diseases are also found in patients without these genetic diseases. For example, mutational analysis has shown the *NF1* and *NF2,* and *p53* tumor suppressor genes are frequently mutated in particular tumors (vestibular schwannomas and meningiomas) in NF2 patients, as well as in their sporadic counterparts.[8] This is true for about one-third of all brain cancer cases. (When a disease is not inherited, it is considered "sporadic." This means that the disease can arise in someone and not be passed on to children. Most cancer cases are sporadic.)

It's interesting to note that patients with other cancers seemingly unrelated to NF2 have also shown mutations in the *NF2* gene. These cancers include neural crest–derived malignant melanomas (a type of skin cancer) and mesotheliomas (cancer of the protective lining of internal organs). This link hints that the *NF2* gene may play a bigger role in the development of cancer than is presently known. Similar to NF2, genetic mutations in the von Hippel–Lindau (*VHL*) tumor suppressor gene occur in not only the hereditary tumors from VHL disease patients but also their sporadic counterparts. The *VHL* gene is significant as a frequently mutated cancer-related gene in sporadic renal cell carcinoma.[7]

Furthermore, 70 percent of families with Li-Fraumeni syndrome have mutations in a key cell regulator (which ensures healthy cell cycle function): the multipurpose *p53* tumor suppressor gene. These mutations stop the p53 regulatory protein from protecting the cell. The job of this regulatory protein, p53, is to stop cells with damaged DNA from dividing, thereby inhibiting tumor development. When this regulatory protein is mutated, it cannot stop damaged cells from replicating. The result can be tumor growth.[17] But healthy people may also have mutations in suppressor genes for other diseases when that disease is not present.

Some studies have shown that mutations in key proteins used for cell detoxification (cytochrome p450 and glutathione) are linked with a higher risk of brain tumors and cancer. Research has also shown that people with genetic mutations affecting oxidative metabolism, immune response, or DNA stability and repair may also have an increased susceptibility to brain cancer and other cancers.[18]

Mutagen Sensitivity

Mutagens, or agents that cause mutations in DNA, do not affect everyone equally. A person's mutagen sensitivity may reflect the effectiveness of DNA repair systems. Or in other words, if DNA is not adequately repaired, it may be more sensitive to mutagens.

Studies suggest that people with lymphocytes especially sensitive to gamma radiation have a higher risk of brain tumors, as well as glioma. This cellular sensitivity to radiation is thought to be due to genetic damage in the DNA repair pathway, although the connection between glioma development and mutagen sensitivity needs further study.[19]

RISK FROM RADIATION

Exposure to Ionizing Radiation

Ionizing radiation has enough energy to break the bonds in DNA structure, causing DNA instability. Exposure to ionizing radiation is consistently associated with an increased risk for brain cancer; even low-dose exposures when they occur over the long term can raise the risk. This is a concern in some workplaces. As an example, researchers found a significant increase in brain cancer risk for nuclear industry workers.[3]

People can be exposed to ionizing radiation in other ways, such as during medical treatments for fungal infections in skin (tinea capitis) or hemangioma (a benign growth) in children or babies. These low-dose treatments are linked to an increased risk of nerve sheath tumors, meningiomas, and gliomas.

Therapeutic ionizing radiation, however, is a strong risk factor for brain cancer. People treated with radiation therapy for lymphoblastic leukemia as children—as well as for other cancers—may be at a higher risk for brain cancer. Adult patients who have had radiation treatments in the nasopharynx area (nasal part of the pharynx), for example, will also have a higher risk for brain cancer. All in all, primary brain tumors develop more often among patients treated with ionizing radiation.

New Uses for Radiation Treatments, and New Risks

As technology advances, new uses for medical radiation have also developed, along with questions about cancer risks. Radiation treatments for nervous system diseases such as intracranial arteriovenous malformation can deliver high doses of radiation to areas of the brain. Computed tomography (CT) scans, including brain scans, are useful and thus increasingly employed. But some research suggests people exposed to medical radiation have a higher risk of nervous system tumors and that the risk continues all their lives, no matter what age they were when they received the radiation.[15]

Atomic Bomb Survivors and Cancer Risk, Dangers of Radiation

Survivors of the atomic bomb that hit Hiroshima had high rates of tumors of the central nervous system and pituitary gland, including meningiomas, shwannomas, gliomas, and pituitary tumors, according to one study.[15] Survivors' cancer rates climbed the closer they had been to the bombing site.

Scientists are not sure how prenatal exposure affects risk, however. Research in Japan has not shown a higher risk for brain cancer or benign brain tumors among those who were exposed to radiation from the atomic bomb in utero.[15] Other research has found prenatal radiation exposure increases risk for child-hood brain tumors 20 to 60 percent. There does not appear to be a higher risk for childhood brain cancers or tumors from parents' radiation exposure before conception.

Cell Phone Use

The safety of cell phone use continues to be a topic of debate. Cell phones emit radiofrequency energy, a form of electromagnetic radiation, and although high levels of this energy can heat—and potentially damage—human tissues, the current research suggests that the amount of radiofrequency energy emitted by mobile phones is too low to heat tissue. More than a dozen studies have exam-ined cell phone use for any connection to brain tumors or brain cancer, and the majority found little or no elevated risk for brain tumors.[14] For more discussion on cell phones and cancer, see chapter 22, "Controversies Regarding Commonly Perceived Risk Factors and Cancer."

HEALTH RISK FACTORS

A Weak Immune System

People with compromised immune systems, such as those with HIV-AIDS infection, may have a higher risk for brain cancer or AIDS-related brain lym-phomas.[4]

Viral Infections

Few epidemiological studies have looked at the connection between viruses and human brain cancer, although research shows that retroviruses, papovavi-ruses, and adenoviruses cause brain tumors (and brain cancer) in animals. Some research suggests a link between mothers who had chicken pox (varicella zoster virus) during pregnancy and children who developed gliomas, but other studies have not found a connection.[9]

Other research focused on herpesviruses and the development of brain tumors but found no link.[10] However, scientists have found evidence that Epstein-Barr virus infection may play a role in brain cancer development in AIDS patients.[11]

More research is needed to learn what role viruses play in human brain cancer development.

Dietary Factors

What we eat may have an impact on our risk for brain cancer, for good or ill. Preserved and smoked meats and fish are generous sources of nitrates and nitrites, chemicals that the human body metabolizes, creating toxic by-products called *N*-nitroso compounds. Experiments on animals have shown these chemicals to be neurocarcinogenic (chemicals that can induce brain cancer). Fried, barbecued, or overly cooked or browned meat can also expose diners to other neurocarcinogens called heterocyclic amines.

These toxic compounds can damage DNA, possibly in developing fetuses as well as adults, and thereby contribute to human brain cancer development. One hypothesis is that adult cancers may develop because of infant or prenatal exposure.[12,20] While a variety of vegetables also contain nitrites, researchers believe vitamins within the food may prevent *N*-nitroso compounds from forming.

Some foods, such as nitrate-rich barbecue meat, may increase brain cancer risk because of the oxidants produced as metabolic by-products. Oxidants are also produced naturally in the body, as by-products of normal aerobic respiration, when cells fight infections (and produce nitric oxide), or as oxidative by-products of the cytochrome p450 detoxification enzyme function. These oxidants can harm DNA; unrepaired DNA damage could over time contribute to brain cancer development.[21]

The remedy for toxic oxidants, of course, is to consume foods rich in antioxidants. These are chemicals that counteract the action of oxidants, removing them or lowering their concentration in the body and thus lessening DNA or cellular damage. Antioxidants may even assist in DNA repair. Antioxidant-rich foods include fruits and vegetables and some vitamin supplements.

However, scientists have not been able to consistently show (through studies of diets and vitamin supplements) that *N*-nitroso compounds, antioxidants, or specific nutrients affect the risk of adult or childhood brain tumors.[12]

Smoking

Researchers have not found consistent data linking tobacco smoke with brain cancer. That said, carcinogenic *N*-nitroso compounds found in tobacco smoke can cross the blood-brain barrier. Some researchers suggest these toxic compounds, along with their harmful metabolic compounds, may contribute to the development of brain tumors. So far, no evidence shows that expectant mothers who smoke are raising their unborn child's risk for brain tumors.[12]

Chemical Exposure at Home

Some studies suggest a link between the use of hair dyes and hair sprays and brain tumors. Most research on chemical exposure in the home has looked at prenatal and postnatal exposures to pesticides (such as household insecticides) and association with childhood brain tumors. Some studies suggest a link between these products and childhood brain cancer.[22,23]

Risk Factors in the Workplace

Some work environments bring employees in contact with harsh occupational or industrial substances that may be neurotoxic (natural or artificial chemicals that are toxic to nerve cells) or carcinogenic. Research shows pesticides can induce brain cancer in animal experiments, while formaldehyde used by embalmers, pathologists, and other professionals seems to increase their risk of brain cancer. Another suspect substance for increasing risk of brain cancer is vinyl chloride, used in manufacturing plastics.

Other possible problem substances include organic solvents, lubricating oils, acrylonitrile, phenols and phenolic compounds, formaldehyde, and polycyclic aromatic hydrocarbons. Some of these substances have produced brain tumors in laboratory animals—although at least one, polycyclic aromatic hydrocarbons, had to be directly implanted in animal brains for tumors to generate, an unlikely scenario for human employees. Worker contact with these substances is likely to be limited to inhalation or contact with skin. Complicating the question, workers are usually exposed to more than one chemical or industrial substance. This can create chemical combinations that may increase or reduce the cancer risk. Because of these complicating factors, even large cohort studies have not been able to find solid links between specific chemicals and human brain tumors or brain cancer—nor for known carcinogens.[12]

Brain Cancer Risk Factors that May Not Cause Brain Cancer

Some noninherited risk factors can be associated with brain cancer but do not have a causative relationship to the disease. These include symptoms such as epilepsy, seizures, and convulsions—all signs that can point medical professionals toward a diagnosis. In the same way, a head injury may not cause a brain tumor, but it may make it more likely that a brain tumor is discovered.

Some studies have associated certain diseases with brain cancer, such as an increased risk for meningioma among colorectal cancer or breast cancer patients. Other research found that people with small cell lung carcinoma were three times as likely to have brain tumors; while patients with adenocarcinoma (cancer of the epithelial cells that line cavities) were twice as likely to have brain tumors. Other risk factors may be the reason for these connections.[12]

SUMMARY

The available research on brain cancer suggests that this disease is the product of a combination of toxic dietary, environmental, or workplace exposures—unless it arises as a result of a rare, hereditary disease. Yet inherited risk factors account for a small proportion of brain cancer cases, less than 10 percent, as discussed above. The disease's prevalence in some families could also be explained by family members' common exposure to harmful agents, as some studies have shown that brain tumors can occur in families without predisposing hereditary diseases.

Lifestyle, workplace, and environmental exposures—many within an individual's control—likely account for the rest.

Chapter 3

Breast Cancer

You probably know someone who has, or who had, breast cancer. After lung cancer it is the most common cause of death by cancer among women. The National Cancer Institute estimates that in 2010 about 207,090 women in the United States developed breast cancer, while about 39,840 women died from the disease.[16]

As other cancers do, breast cancer takes its name from the main location where it is found—in the breast area. Often the cancer forms in milk ducts in the nipple or in the glands that make milk (lobules), but this cancer can form in any tissues of the breast.

A woman's chances of getting breast cancer increase as she ages, and most women who get breast cancer are over age 60. A woman's chances also rise if she has a family history of breast cancer, especially if her mother, sister, or daughter is diagnosed with the disease. And if a woman has breast cancer in one breast, her chances of having the disease in the other breast increase. As the vast majority of breast cancer patients are women, this chapter will have a female focus. But men also get breast cancer.

BREAST CANCER AND MEN

Breast cancer in men is rare, representing less than 1 percent of cases. This means about 1,970 U.S. men developed breast cancer in 2010, according to the National Cancer Institute. That same year, an estimated 390 men in the United States died from this disease.[16]

Some of the risk factors are the same for men as for women, such as a higher risk of breast cancer if a relative has the disease—especially a close relative such as a sibling or parent. Exposure to radiation can increase breast cancer risk for men, as can hormonal imbalances and an inherited gene mutation (*BRCA2*) that will be discussed later in this chapter.[10]

Men with breast cancer tend to be between the ages of 60 and 70, although this cancer can develop at any age. Men's survival rates are similar to women's; however, men tend to get diagnosed at a later stage, so they often have a worse prognosis.

Symptoms

Breast cancer may be caught in its early stages by those who know their breast areas through self-examination. Things to look for include a lump or a thickening in the breast or underarm area, nipple tenderness or discharge, a nipple that becomes inverted, or breast-area skin or a nipple that becomes red, scaly, or swollen.

This disease is often not painful in the early stages. Still, anyone with breast pain or other symptoms that persist should consult a doctor. In most cases, these symptoms are caused by other health problems and are not due to cancer.

RISK FACTORS

Ethnicity

Breast cancer is a complicated disease. The term "breast cancer" covers a variety of diseases found in the breast. Scientists call this grouping of diseases "recognized biological subtypes." Confounding attempts to understand breast cancer is the fact that different clinical outcomes are often connected to ethnicity.

African American women typically have higher-grade (more aggressive), later-stage diagnoses. These patients also have a lower survival rate. Ethnicity and socioeconomic factors may affect access to screening and treatment and thus survival rate. But researchers have found important differences in the cancer diseases between women of different ethnicities independent of such considerations.

Despite Caucasian women being diagnosed with breast cancer more often than Latina, Asian, or African American women,[8] African American women have the highest rates of premenopausal breast cancer. Across all age groups, Asian women have lower breast cancer rates.

While African American women face the highest risk for developing breast cancer before age 50, they also have an increased risk of having more aggressive forms of breast cancer with higher-grade tumors that are steroid hormone receptor negative. Many factors could play a role in the vulnerability of African American women to breast cancer, but some studies suggest genetic variation in certain genes may be the key.[11] It is interesting to note that although Asian American women have lower breast cancer incidence compared with other U.S. women, Asian American women's breast cancer rates catch up to those of Caucasian women after several generations in the United States. This indicates that diet, the environment, or another influence in the United States may increase vulnerability to breast cancer.[12]

Reproductive and Hormonal Risk Factors

Breast cancer is linked to reproductive and hormonal factors.[1] Postmenopausal women with relatively high serum (clear liquid separate from clotted blood) concentrations of sex hormones have nearly double the risk for this disease compared to women of the same age with lower concentrations of these hormones.

Another clue implicating hormonal influence is that women who take estrogen plus progestin to treat the symptoms of menopause seem to increase their risk of breast cancer.

A longer reproductive period appears to add to risk as well. Research has shown that women with an early onset of menstruation (before age 12) or a late start of menopause (after age 55) also have a higher risk for breast cancer. Not having children amplifies a woman's risk for this disease. According to several large studies, there is no connection between breast cancer risk and abortion or miscarriage.[2]

Menopause

Scientists have been looking at why menopause appears to be such a critical time for breast cancer development. A key change that occurs at menopause is the response of estrogen receptors (ERs). As estrogen needs these receptors to carry out its hormone functions in the body, the incidence of breast cancer may be different depending on the estrogen receptor status of tumors (if tumor growth depends on an estrogen receptor). Scientific studies indicate that menopause exerts a greater protective effect on estrogen-receptor negative (ER–) breast cancer than on estrogen-receptor positive (ER+) breast cancer.

Tumor status is important as, for example, a tumor can become ER negative and therefore no longer express (manifest) the estrogen receptor. This is a key concept, as most breast cancers are treated with antihormones. If a patient has an ER negative tumor, the antiestrogens will not have any effect.

For both Caucasian and African American women, the age-specific rates of ER-negative breast cancer stop increasing after age 50, but age-specific rates of ER-positive breast cancer continue to increase after 50.[7] Studies have shown that younger age at onset is associated with more undifferentiated tumor types and low ER content.

Family History and Inherited Disposition

Family history is one of the strongest risk factors for breast cancer. If a woman has a close relative, such as a mother, sister, or daughter with breast cancer, her risk rises;

if this relative developed the disease before age 40, the woman's risk is at the highest. Women may also face an increased risk of breast cancer if they have other relatives with the disease, in either their mother's or father's families. A person's chances of getting breast cancer also increase if she is of Jewish ancestry, or if she or a family member has had ovarian cancer, or if a relative has had bilateral breast cancer.

Currently, scientists believe two primary mutated genes are linked to a risk for breast cancer. These are known as *BRCA*1 and *BRCA*2. These mutated genes were discovered during studies of families with several generations of members diagnosed with breast cancer. Both genes encode proteins that researchers believe are responsible for repairing damaged DNA, among other actions. A damaged system for repairing DNA makes a person more vulnerable to cancer. The *BRCA*1 and *BRCA*2 mutations have also been linked with ovarian cancer. People from an Ashkenazi Jewish background are more likely to have these mutations. Women can determine their risk for these damaged genes by drawing up a detailed family history or undergoing genetic counseling. It may be important to test for these mutations in some women.[6]

Although family history is a key risk factor for breast cancer, one should note that less than 10 percent of cases can be linked to hereditary gene mutations such as *BRCA*1 or *BRCA*2.[5] These inheritable mutations account for only a small number of cases, even within a family cluster of breast cancer patients. These mutations are often absent in sporadic breast cancer cases.

Radiation Exposure

Women (and men) who receive radiation therapy to the chest and breast area before age 30 have a higher risk for breast cancer. In fact, the younger a patient is when she is treated with radiation, the higher her risk of breast cancer in her later years.[3] Patients treated with radiation for Hodgkin lymphoma are an example of a higher risk group for breast cancer.

CHEMICAL EXPOSURE

Pesticides and other harsh chemicals may increase breast cancer risk. Some people are more vulnerable to chemical carcinogens and thus likely to develop cancer. These people may have proactive enzymes that increase the production of procarcinogens (compounds that become carcinogenic after the body metabolizes them), or they may have defective enzymes that are incapable of detoxifying hazardous carcinogenic intermediates from environmental chemicals. This would give them a higher risk for breast cancer.[4]

Breast Tissue Type, Fitness, and Breast Cancer Risk

Women with dense or fatty breast tissue may be at a higher risk for breast cancer, as are women who are overweight or obese after menopause. Physical inactivity, especially as a lifestyle habit, also increases breast cancer risk.[13]

Diet, Alcohol, and Breast Cancer Risk

Plenty of research shows that what people eat can have a preventive or caus-ative effect on a variety of cancers, including breast cancer. For example, scien-tists believe deficiencies in micronutrients such as the B vitamin folate (folic acid) can negatively influence cells' ability to repair DNA.[14]

Meanwhile, studies show that women who drink alcohol can increase their risk for breast cancer, especially if they have a low folate intake.[9] Therefore, a diet sufficient in folate and low in alcohol is important to decrease one's chances of getting breast cancer.

Scientists are gathering other evidence that suggests that, in general, folate inadequacy may be a key risk factor for an assortment of cancer types. Their research shows that low folate intake and status in the body are positively linked with a whole list of cancers, such as cervical, lung, esophageal, pancreatic, and in particular, colorectal cancer.

High folate consumption also appears to offer protective benefits against postmenopausal breast cancer and is especially beneficial for women who have a moderate to high alcohol consumption. Chapter 17, "Nutrition and Cancer," has more discussion on the connections between diet and breast cancer.

Smoking

Cigarette smoke is full of carcinogens. As tobacco smoke causes or is linked to several different types of cancers, it's possible this toxic substance may also affect breast cancer risk.[15]

An Important Note on Risk Factors

Most women with these risk factors do not develop breast cancer. In fact, most breast cancer patients do not have a family history of the disease or any clear risk factors, with the possible exception of aging.

SUMMARY

While science still has much to learn about breast cancer, biological differ-ences between cancers may be due to environmental exposures, genetics, lifestyle choices, or nutritional habits of patients.

Women (and men) can reduce their chances of getting this disease by avoiding known risk factors. Recommended lifestyle adjustments include eating a nutrient-rich diet, exercising, losing excess body weight, avoiding moderate to excessive alcohol consumption, and quitting smoking.

Not all risk factors can be avoided, however. Some people may have a pre-disposition for breast cancer, either through inherited mutated genes or because they have had breast cancer before. In such cases, it may be prudent for these women to discuss with their doctors the pros and cons of starting mammography screening early as well as having breast ultrasounds, magnetic resonance imaging (MRI) examinations, or more frequent breast examinations.

Many health organizations, such as the American Cancer Society, continue to recommend that women in their 20s and 30s have a clinical breast examination once every three years and that average-risk women age 40 and older have a yearly exam as well as annual mammograms. They also advise self-check examinations. It should be noted here that some medical professionals have recommended changes to screening practice, including that average-risk women not have mammograms until they reach age 50. See chapter 20 for more on the screening debate.

The good news about breast cancer is that it often can be successfully treated; the past 25 years have seen huge leaps forward in the medical management of breast cancer.

Chapter 4

Cervical Cancer

Cervical cancer is one of the deadliest cancers among women, especially for those who cannot afford the cost of a Pap smear test. While cervical cancer is usually a slow-growing cancer, it often will not have symptoms in its early stages. A regular Pap smear screening is essential for early detection of this disease and the best opportunity for treatment. But many women in poorer regions of the world are not able to afford this test.

In 2010 an estimated 553,000 women from around the world were diagnosed with cervical cancer, and about 288,000 died from the disease, according to the International Agency for Research on Cancer.[16]

Yet this disease is one of best understood forms of cancer. Scientists have learned that the common human papillomavirus (HPV)—a type of sexually transmitted disease[2]—is the cause of nearly all cases of cervical cancer.[1]

The connection between cervical cancer and sexual activity has been known for some time. Dr. Dr. Rigoni-Stern noticed in 1842 that, while Italian nuns rarely had cervical cancer, prostitutes were particularly vulnerable to the disease.[3] He reasoned that women with multiple sexual partners had an increased risk for cervical cancer. And having sexual partners who themselves have many sexual partners also increases women's risk for the disease, most likely because this increases their chances for catching HPV.

THE HUMAN PAPILLOMAVIRUS

First identified in cervical tissue in 1974, this group of viruses has more than 100 different types and has been linked to cancers of the anus, vulva, vagina, and penis. Some HPVs are low risk, such as HPV6 and HPV11, which are usually responsible only for noncancerous genital warts. Researchers have learned that only 15 HPV types typically cause cancer, with HPV16 as the most pervasive: this virus is found in more than 99 percent of all patients with cervical cancer.[11]

Research has shown that HPV causes cancer by ultimately affecting two important genes, known as *Rb* and *p53*. These genes encode for proteins that prevent cells with damaged DNA from dividing and help repair or eliminate the injured cells. This process helps prevent tumor growth.

HPV corrupts this process and pirates a cell's regenerative abilities by incorporating its own genetic material into the host cell, forcing the cell to produce more viruses. At the same time, the human cell can no longer regulate the Rb and p53 proteins,[4] leaving the person vulnerable to tumor growth.

HPV: A Sexually Transmitted Disease, Most of the Time

People become infected with HPV through sexual activity, so all who are sexually active risk exposure to this disease. Yet some of these viruses have infected women who have never had sexual intercourse, and according to one study, virgins have an HPV infection rate of 14.8 percent. This viral infection appears to be passed from mothers to their children during childbirth.[5,12]

A commonplace disease, nearly all cervical HPV infections disappear within a year or two. Most of the viruses are relatively harmless—it is the persistent HPV16 infection that triggers the majority of cervical cancer cases. The disease tends to be diagnosed about 20 years following infection, although the infection itself can appear after a woman's first experience of sexual intercourse. Researchers theorize that the friction of sexual activity activates the virus.

Symptoms

The symptoms for cervical cancer resemble symptoms for several other conditions, so it is essential women check with their doctors if they have any concerns. Commonly, women with cervical cancer will experience abnormal vaginal bleeding. This may include bleeding between menstrual periods, having longer and heavier periods, and bleeding after sexual intercourse and after menopause. Women may also experience more vaginal discharge and pain during sexual intercourse.

Early Detection

From the time of its development in the early 20th century the Papanicolaou cervical cytology screening, or Pap smear, has become the standard method of screening for cervical cancer. This test helps prevent the disease by catching it in its early stages through identification of precancerous cells or other cervical cell changes. As precancerous cells can be treated before they become cancerous, regular Pap smears are important to women's health. It follows that women who do not undergo regular Pap tests have an increased risk for cervical cancer.

The Multifaceted Development of Cervical Cancer

While high-risk HPVs can be found in more than 99 percent of all cervical cancers, in fact only a few women infected with these high-risk HPVs get cervical cancer. This tells researchers that other factors play a role in producing the disease, and the very few cases of cervical cancer that are not linked to this virus support this idea. Scientists have looked at vaginal douching, use of birth control pills, infection with herpes simplex virus type 2, and nutrition as contributing factors.[13]

Studies have shown that women with HPV infections who smoke cigarettes have a higher risk of cervical cancer compared to nonsmoking women with HPV infections. Other research suggests that tissues infected with high-risk HPVs, namely, HPV16 or HPV18, and exposed to tar can produce cervical cancer.[6] Scientists believe toxic tars from tobacco smoke or other sources likely find their way to the cervix through the bloodstream. The smoke contains more than 4,000 compounds, 16 of which are known human carcinogens, such as benzoapyrene polycyclic aromatic amines, and tobacco-specific nitrosamines. Some research shows that the cervical mucus of female smokers has three times the amount of tobacco-specific nitrosamines as that of nonsmoking women.[7]

Women may also be exposed to tars through inhaling smoke from wood and coal-burning stoves or through the use of tar-based vaginal douches. Other risk factors linked with cervical cancers include a past *Chlamydia* infection (another sexually transmitted disease) and excessive alcohol consumption.[13]

Women who use steroid hormones may also raise their chances of getting cervical cancer, according to a large multinational study. The long-term use of birth control pills is thought to increase the risk for this disease, and much more so when these women are also infected with HPV; their risk climbs fourfold.[8] Women with weakened immune systems, such as those who have HIV-AIDS or who use drugs that depress the immune system, are also at a higher risk for cervical cancer. As with other cancers, aging is a risk factor for cervical cancers. Most women who get this disease are over 40.

HPV and Other Cancer Sites

Scientists do not know yet if an anal HPV infection can lead to cervical cancer. HPV infection in the anus is found frequently among women and men with HIV and who have compromised immune systems. Some research suggests that anal HPV may also be relatively common among healthy women, in much the same way that cervical HPV infection is prevalent. About 13 percent of women have infections at both locations. While the viral infection may be transmitted to the anus through sexual activity, such as anal intercourse, some scientists have proposed that HPV can be spread by nonsexual means. HPV in vaginal discharge, for example, could be easily passed to the nearby anus. This poses a health risk. Research has determined that HPV can be found in up to 90 percent of anal tumors from men and women. Anal cancer cases have increased in the past 20 years across gender lines in the United States, and some evidence shows HPV-triggered cancers in the anus show a development similar to cancers in the cervix: first viral infection, then lesions, followed by cancer.[9]

HPV Vaccine and Cervical Cancer Prevention

Women have two options when it comes to cervical cancer prevention. For decades, the Pap smear test has had an enormous impact on women's health by making it possible to catch precancerous and cancerous cells in their early stages. Organized national screening programs in the United States and other countries have helped reduce the number of cervical cancer cases.[14] Although frequent Pap testing is essential for abnormal changes to be caught, this is a costly process. Researchers have sought less expensive options—some focusing on the link between HPV infection and cervical cancer. And so the HPV vaccine was developed.

While not all HPV infections cause cancer, nearly all cases of cervical cancer are triggered by HPV infection with 1 of the 15 most carcinogenic types. The most deadly is HPV16, trailed by types 18 and 31.

As noted, many women will contract at least one HPV infection in their lifetime. And most will not develop cervical cancer, thanks to their immune systems. But as nearly all cases of cervical cancer can be attributed to infection with either of the two highest-risk viral infections (HPV16 and HPV18), scientists have formulated a vaccine to combat these infections.

The HPV vaccine could have a global impact on the incidence on cervical cancer. It is also highly controversial as it works on women only if they have not yet been infected with HPV. This means the vaccine should be administered before sexual activity begins, perhaps even in childhood.

The first vaccine on the market, Merck's Gardasil, was designed to prevent cervical cancer, precancerous genital lesions, and genital warts from infections by HPV types 6, 11, 16, and 18. HPV types 16 and 18 are linked to about 70 percent of these cancers, while HPV types 6 and 11 generate about 90 percent of genital warts. Gardasil was tested on girls and women ages 9 to 26, and was licensed by the Food and Drug Administration in 2006. This vaccine offers no benefits to anyone already infected with HPV. A review prepared for the FDA in 2009 noted that the vaccine could also be given to boys and men aged 9 to 26 to prevent genital warts.[15]

The vaccine is administered through three injections within six months. It works as other vaccines against viral infections, in that the vaccine stimulates the body to create antibodies to prevent infection and cervical cancer development. This HPV vaccine does not protect against the more unusual forms of HPV, and so even vaccinated women should continue to have regular Pap tests.

Although some in the United States have argued that the vaccine should be mandatory, others believe it should be up to parents whether their daughters are vaccinated. Some of the controversy centers on teen sexuality and that, for girls to be vaccinated, parents would need to tell them about the vaccine's purpose. Some have suggested that girls who are vaccinated may believe that sex is now safe for them—a fallacy, as HPV infection risk increases with the number of sexual partners.

SUMMARY

Cervical cancer is a well-understood disease, thanks to the discovery of its connection to HPV infection. It's also one of the most preventable human cancers. It has identifiable early signs, develops slowly and can be treated successfully.[10] This means that with effective preventive screening, it is possible to catch the disease at its earliest stages.

Women should note that precancerous cervical changes and early cancer formation in the cervix often are not painful or otherwise symptomatic. Therefore women should see their doctors for routine Pap tests to catch any early changes in their cervical tissues. This gives them the best chance to have precancerous tumors treated before cancer develops.

While the HPV vaccine can be an effective tool against a carcinogenic viral infection, the vaccine protects against only particular virus types and should be administered before HPV exposure. Vaccinated women should continue to have regular Pap test screening to check for rare but harmful HPV infections.

Chapter 5

Colorectal Cancer

It may be the fourth-most-common cause of death by cancer in the United States—killing an estimated 51,000 people in 2010—but colorectal cancer is also the most preventable form of cancer death, if caught in its early stages.[13]

The term *colorectal cancer* refers to cancer diseases that develop in either the colon, the long part of the large intestine, or the rectum, the last few inches of the intestine leading to the anus. It is sometimes called large-bowel cancer. The cancers that typically form in these areas are adenocarinomas, beginning in the mucous-forming cells.[9] This cancer appears to be highest in developed countries: it's associated with obesity and a sedentary lifestyle.[10]

SYMPTOMS

Symptoms may not be apparent in the disease's earliest stages. As the cancer develops, however, one may note a wide variety of symptoms such as diarrhea or constipation, a feeling of fullness in the bowel even after elimination, and blood (vivid red or dark) in stool, which may be narrower than normal. Unexplained weight loss, fatigue, gas, bloating, cramps, and nausea are also common symptoms. It is important to note that other health problems besides colorectal cancer may cause these symptoms, but a doctor should be consulted to rule out this disease. A colonoscopy may be recommended to look for abnormalities in the colon, such as polyps (benign growths that may lead to cancer).

RISK FACTORS

Age is one of the biggest risk factors for colorectal cancer, particularly as one passes age 50; 60 is the mean age of diagnosis. Other major risk factors include having parents or siblings with the disease (especially at a young age) or, for women, having a history of ovarian, uterine, or breast cancer. People with ulcerative colitis, Crohn disease, or other chronic colon inflammation will have a higher risk of developing colorectal cancer. An unhealthy diet lacking in essential nutrients, smoking tobacco, and drinking excessive amounts of alcohol can also increase one's colorectal cancer risk, as can a sedentary lifestyle. These factors are discussed in more depth later in this chapter.

Family History and Hereditary Risk Factors

As noted above, people with siblings or parents or many close relatives with colorectal cancer have a higher risk for this disease. A family's predisposition can be due to inheritable gene mutations that make family members more vulnerable. However, research shows these cases likely amount to less than 10 percent of all colorectal cancer cases.[2]

Hereditary Nonpolyposis Colorectal Cancer

Hereditary nonpolyposis colorectal cancer (HNPCC, also known as Lynch syndrome) is the most frequently seen of these rare, inherited conditions. This type of colon cancer is caused by germ-line mutations in DNA mismatch repair (*MMR*) genes. *MMR* genes help repair genetic material and fix mistakes in DNA replication, essential services to the health of cells. Colorectal cells that have a hindered repair system are more prone to genetic damage and, as a result, are more at risk for developing colorectal cancer.[3]

It is an unfortunate fact that the majority of people with the *HNPCC* mutation will develop colon cancer, typically at about age 44. People with this syndrome may also develop other cancers, often in the stomach, urinary tract, or endometrium.

Familial Adenomatous Polyposis

Familial adenomatous polyposis (FAP) is an inherited condition that causes hundreds of polyps (or tumors) to grow on the inner walls of the colon and rectum, and it can lead to colon cancer. The polyps can start growing during a person's youth but tend to appear in people older than 50. While the polyps are usually noncancerous, a prophylactic colectomy (surgery to remove any amount of the colon as a preventive measure) should be done, otherwise these growths could become malignant. Untreated, people with this condition tend to develop cancer at age 44—at least two decades earlier than people without this syndrome tend to develop colorectal cancer.[11]

Like HNPCC, gene mutations cause FAP. In this case the changes are found in the adenomatous polyposis coli gene, another player in tumor suppression. This gene also encodes for an important protein that helps regulate dividing cells and stop damaged DNA from getting passed on. This is a rare deviation, however. It's thought that people with FAP amount to less than 1 percent of colorectal cancer patients.

Chronic Colon Inflammation

People with ulcerative colitis, Crohn disease, or other chronic colon inflam-mation have a higher risk of developing colorectal cancer. Chronic inflammation may be due to persistent bacterial infection (which kills protective cells lining the colon, resulting in sores and ulcers). The immune system may cause chronic inflammation as a result of reacting abnormally to infection.

Diet

An unhealthy lifestyle puts one at a higher risk for colorectal cancer, particu-larly a typical Western diet that's high in animal fat and low in fiber, fruit, and vegetables.[4] The opposite is also true: studies show that people who eat plenty of fruit and raw and green vegetables—particularly cruciferous vegetables such as broccoli—have a decreased risk for colorectal cancer. This is because of the special twofold protective function of fiber in the bowel. First of all, fiber is bulky and helps keep waste moving quickly through the body—therefore helping elimi-nate toxins efficiently. Secondly, as it ferments, fiber creates short-chain fatty acids (one is butyrate) that soothe inflammation and prevent cancer formation, boosting the colon's defenses and easing oxidative stress.[5]

Vegetables, too, play a role in fighting colorectal cancer thanks to the action of their micronutrients. For example, carotenoids are antioxidants that deactivate toxins and carcinogens, while bioactive agents such as flavonoids or phenols have powerful anticancerous effects, inhibiting DNA damage caused by toxins. Found in vegetables, folate is thought to have protective effects, as do vitamin D, vitamin E, and complex carbohydrates in general. The micronutrients ingested through food sources are thought to be absorbed best by the body.

Meanwhile, frequently eating large amounts of eggs and sugar can increase your risk for this disease. Some research shows that eating well-done meat also raises the risk as does meat or fish cooked at high temperatures. High heat pro-duces the carcinogens heterocyclic amine and nitrosamines; studies on laboratory animals demonstrate that these compounds can trigger colon tumors.[14]

Calcium

Some studies show that taking calcium supplements can reduce your risk for colon cancer; others demonstrate calcium's ability to protect against cancer re-currence. Calcium benefits the body by binding fatty acids and bile in the bowel, an action that limits the contact of these possible carcinogens with the lining of the colon.[6] More information on food supplements and cancer is covered in chapter 21.

Exercise

Numerous studies show that regular exercise reduces cancer risk, especially for colorectal cancer.[7] Some researchers believe these benefits are because exercise stimulates colonic movement (peristalsis), thus keeping waste products in motion through the colon and limiting the organ lining's contact with toxins.

Exercise also has immediate and long-term positive hormonal effects on the body's immune system and contributes to a balanced metabolism, particularly in lean people. This means lower insulin, triacylglycerol, and glucose levels. These factors may inhibit tumor growth, particularly that of colorectal cancer.[1]

Alcohol

Research shows a stronger association between high alcohol consumption and colorectal cancer in men than in women. This is likely because women tend to consume less alcohol.[1] Some studies indicate that the cancer risk is due to total ethanol (the active component in alcoholic beverages) consumption, rather than any specific kind of drink. Researchers suspect that ethanol acts as a solvent or otherwise has a cytotoxic effect (or damaging effect on cells) in tissues in the colon or in the upper alimentary tract. One reason may be that the acetaldehyde in alcohol attaches to DNA and damages genetic material, as it is already known that alcohol hinders DNA repair. People who drink alcohol excessively also tend to have nutrient deficiencies, such as lower folate, which may add to its damaging effects.[12]

Smoking

The most preventable risk factor, smoking tobacco, is linked to a whole host of cancers throughout the body, such as lung, stomach, esophagus, bladder, kidney, pancreas, and colorectal cancer. The smoke contains carcinogenic compounds such as heterocyclic amines, aromatic amines, nitrosamines, and aromatic hydrocarbons. These toxins reach the colon via the circulatory system or the alimentary tract and may seriously harm or deform key genes that protect the body from cancer.[8]

SUMMARY

No one knows the exact cause of most cases of colorectal cancer, but research shows the best way to protect oneself from this disease is to eat a diet rich in fiber, fruit, and vegetables and exercise regularly. If necessary, use nonsteroidal anti-inflammatory drugs (NSAIDs).[1] Studies have shown that people who used these over-the-counter drugs for other symptoms such as arthritis have lower risks for colorectal cancer. However, note that some of these products can have worrisome side effects, such as irritated or bleeding stomach. Therefore health experts do not recommend NSAIDs as a preventive strategy for people at average risk for colorectal cancer.

If you have colorectal cancer, you may be concerned that family members will also develop the disease. People who may be at risk should talk to their doctor regarding screening; relatives of those with HNPCC or FAP can undergo genetic testing to check for specific genetic mutations.

Chapter 6

Esophageal Cancer

Esophageal cancer strikes the passageway between the mouth and stomach and can be easily missed in its early stages, a sad fact that accounts for it being the sixth-most-common means of death by cancer. In 2010 an estimated 507,000 people worldwide were diagnosed with esophageal cancer, while 428,000 died from the disease, according to statistics from the International Agency for Research on Cancer.[11] As the numbers show, survival rates for this disease are grim. The scientific data reveals that only one-fifth of patients with this disease will live more than three years past their diagnosis date, while only about 14 percent live to five years after diagnosis.

Part of the reason why this cancer can be so deadly is that by the time most people have experienced the typical first symptom, which is having difficulty swallowing (dysphagia), the cancer has already advanced. This is because the tumors can grow and multiply down the esophageal passageway for some time before disrupting the organ's normal function.

Esophageal cancer is not a common cancer in North America, amounting to only about 1 percent of all cancer diagnoses in the United States. This translates into 16,640 new diagnoses in this country annually (estimates for 2010), with about 14,500 deaths.[19]

SYMPTOMS

The most common first symptoms of this disease are trouble swallowing solid food and the resulting weight loss. These are experienced by about 90 percent of those with this disease. Esophageal cancer patients may also indicate a specific location in their chest or neck where they can feel an obstruction. Unfortunately, as noted previously, a problem with swallowing can be a sign of advanced cancer.

Other symptoms can include back pain, chest pain, heartburn, a hoarse voice or persistent cough, weight loss, and food sticking in the throat. These symptoms, however, can also indicate health problems other than esophageal cancer. Anyone who experiences these symptoms should see a doctor as soon as possible.

RISK FACTORS

Esophageal cancer is much more prevalent in Africa and what some refer to as the "Asian esophageal belt," an area stretching from east Iran to Turkmenistan, Tajikistan, Uzbekistan, Kyrgyzstan, and China (see the discussion on diet, below, for more details).[12] In these high-incidence locations the disease strikes men and women equally, but elsewhere men have a higher risk.

Some research shows that particular families are more prone to this cancer. People who have parents or siblings with the disease have 10 times the risk—although no higher risk has been linked to having distant relatives with esophageal cancer. Someone with a family history of other cancers will have a higher chance of getting esophageal cancer, particularly if those cancers are in the upper gastrointestinal tract, the head, or the neck.[1] This topic is further discussed later in this chapter.

As with many types of cancer, age is a risk factor for esophageal cancer. Most people diagnosed with the disease are older than age 60. Again, a quartet of avoidable lifestyle risk factors for most cancers also applies here: tobacco smoke, excessive alcohol consumption, micronutrient deficiency, and DNA-damaging carcinogens as a result of a poor diet can all increase a person's risk for this disease. It's likely, however, that a combination of risk factors creates a greater risk for this disease.

GENETIC AND HEREDITARY RISK FACTORS

Barrett Esophagus

A precancerous condition called Barrett esophagus is not considered hereditary but may involve some genetic factors.[20] This disease arises after long-term, acid-reflux-induced irritation to the esophagus (when stomach acid is pushed up the esophagus). During acid reflux, glandular cells from the lower areas of the esophagus can replace the squamous (scalelike) cells that normally line the tubular organ's walls and "burn" the esophagus. Barrett esophagus accounts for about 10 percent of esophageal cancer cases. This problem can be compounded if the stomach acid also contains carcinogens, such as tobacco-specific nitrosamines.[3] In any case, suffering from near-daily heartburn can increase risk by up to 43 times for esophageal cancer. Thus avoiding food or drink that relaxes the esophageal sphincter (the muscle that closes the opening to the stomach) and thereby promotes acid reflux is a key to prevention for Barrett esophagus. These include fatty foods, alcohol, dairy products, mints, caffeinated or carbonated drinks, chocolate, citrus fruits, and tomatoes.

Tylosis Syndrome

The only genetic disease known to make a person more prone to esophageal cancer is tylosis syndrome, a condition that causes thickening (hyperkeratosis) of the palms and the soles. Researchers have learned that deletion or mutation of the gene responsible for this has a connection to esophageal cancer. This can be inherited or can be sporadic (that is, it happens in the individual but is not passed on).[4]

Achalasia of the Esophagus

People with achalasia of the esophagus, an apparently hereditary condition (studies have found twin siblings with achalasia of the esophagus),[13] do not have normal movement or peristalsis in their esophagus. This allows food to accumulate at the low end of the organ, and the esophageal sphincter may also not operate normally. This may mean that glandular cells may replace the squamous cells lining lower areas of the esophagus, leading to constant irritation and a higher susceptibility for cancer.

Plummer-Vinson Syndrome

People with Plummer-Vinson syndrome, a hereditary disorder, have difficulty swallowing and are at higher risk for developing squamous cell carcinoma of the esophagus and the mouth.

DNA Repair Mechanism Damage

Research has shown that flaws in key areas of cellular activity can raise the risk for esophageal cancer. These important areas include the functioning of genes responsible for DNA repair and the metabolism of carcinogens. For example, defects in the *BRCA*2 gene, which encodes for DNA repair proteins, have been shown to increase vulnerability to familial esophageal cancer.[5,14]

Mutations in Detoxifying Enzymes

A higher risk of esophageal cancer is also related to damage or deficiencies in genes meant to disarm carcinogens (called phase I and II enzymes). Examples of these types of enzymes include the phase I cytochrome *p*450 enzyme superfamily (a group of genes similar in function or structure) and the phase II glutathione *S*-transferases and *N*-acetyltransferases. Phase II enzymes mainly detoxify chemical toxins.

Mutations and Genomic Instability

Other enzyme defects can lead to precancerous conditions in the esophagus. One is a mutation in the enzyme methylenetetrahydrofolate reductase (*MTHFR*), a key player in folate processing. People with a particular *MTHFR* defect have less folate but higher homocysteine levels in their plasma, a scenario that raises the risk for esophageal cancer. A person with multiple mutations in these important areas of cell function will have less genomic stability. This may mean a higher risk for esophageal cancer, especially if the person is exposed to carcinogens in the environment.[5]

LIFESTYLE FACTORS

Diet: The Major Cancer Risk from Fermented, Salted, or Smoked Foods

Studies have shown that eating some preserved foods can increase the risk for esophageal cancer. Many of these are common to the "Asian esophageal belt" mentioned earlier and include pickled vegetables or the fermented corn often eaten in Transkei-area South Africa, for example. Scientists believe the higher risk may be due to cancer-causing nitrosamines as well as fungal contaminants. Researchers have found high amounts of crop toxins (fusarium mycotoxins) in poorly stored crops or aged corn products from areas of high esophageal cancer concentration.[21,22]

Salted, preserved fish is a commonly consumed food that contributes to esophageal cancer risk in southern China. Smoked meat or fish is also thought to increase risk for this cancer. The culprits are likely the metabolic byproducts of these foods, including carcinogens such as polycyclic aromatic hydrocarbons (PAHs) and nitrosamines. Meat or fish cooked at high temperatures may also contain these toxins.[6]

Some foods can make you sick, while others protect. A number of published studies suggest that people who eat plenty of fruit and vegetables have a lower risk of esophageal cancer as well as other types of cancer. The protective factors may be the vitamins and minerals found in these foods, as research has shown that places with high levels of esophageal cancer incidence tend to have diets low in B vitamins.[5]

The B vitamins riboflavin and niacin are of particular interest. Laboratory research has shown that a lack of riboflavin can trigger esophageal cancer in baboons, while esophageal cancer development was inhibited in laboratory rats that received supplements of riboflavin, niacin, zinc, magnesium, and molybdenum.[15] Esophageal cancer is also linked to diets insufficient in retinol, beta-carotene, riboflavin, vitamin C, and vitamin E. It is not completely understood how vitamins or minerals do their protective work, but vitamins have antioxidant properties and these may help protect cells' DNA from the damaging effects of oxygen free radicals.

Vitamins and minerals may also help prevent the potent carcinogenic N-nitroso compounds from forming. Laboratory animal studies indicate these toxins may play a role in human stomach and esophageal cancers. Some evidence suggests that beta-carotene, vitamin E, and selenium may assist the immune system in ways that hinder cancer processes in the esophagus.[7]

More discussion on the benefits as well as the controversies regarding dietary supplementations is in chapters 17 and 20.

Alcohol and Risk

Research has shown a strong connection between chronic alcohol consumption and esophageal cancer. The reason is that the more alcohol a person drinks, the more this person is exposed to acetaldehyde, the main metabolite of alcohol and a carcinogen.

In most people, the exposure is relatively short, as enzymes process the alcohol to acetaldehyde and then to carbon dioxide and water. The enzymes responsible for these processes are alcohol dehydrogenase (ADH2) and acetaldehyde dehydrogenase (ALDH2). Some people have genetic variants of these enzymes, and their blood-acetaldehyde levels after imbibing vary accordingly. While these *ALDH2* and *ADH2* gene mutations are rare in the West, they are fairly common in China, Korea, Thailand, and Japan. The gene variations give them blood-acetaldehyde concentrations 13 times that of people without the mutations.[16]

When people with the *ALDH2* gene mutation drink alcohol, their faces will flush red and they will feel nauseated, become drowsy, and develop a headache. People with these symptoms should limit or avoid alcohol in their diets. The mutations inhibit their bodies from eliminating the carcinogen acetyladehyde, which increases their risk for esophageal cancer when they drink alcohol.[8]

Opium, Areca Nut, and Tobacco

The elevated esophageal cancer rates across the Asian esophageal belt are due to more than dietary factors. Several habits known to this region can also play a role in the incidence of this disease. For example, opium use, consumption of *soukhteh* (an opium residue), and chewing *nass* (tobacco with lime and ash), as practiced in parts of northeast Iran, are linked to the higher rates of esophageal cancer in those areas.[9]

In Taiwan and other areas in southern Asia, some people habitually chew areca nut (a mild stimulant). These nuts contain high levels of safrole, a DNA-damaging carcinogen that has induced esophageal cancer in laboratory experiments with animals.[17]

Polycyclic aromatic hydrocarbons (PAHs) from tobacco and other sources are also thought to contribute to esophageal cancer incidence. These toxic compounds may be absorbed from inhaling tobacco smoke or eating charred meat, or they may be absorbed from breathing air or consuming food contaminated with smoke from coal burned in unvented stoves. Researchers have found evidence of PAH contamination in esophagectomy (surgery to remove part of the esophagus) samples.[18]

High levels of 1-hydroxy pyrene (a metabolite of benzoapyrene, a form of PAH) have also been found in urine samples of people with a high risk of PAH contamination exposure, showing that the toxin is indeed being taken into the body.

The evidence suggests that decreasing exposure to PAH contamination may lower the risk of esophageal cancer.

OCCUPATIONAL RISK FACTORS

Depending on their work environments, it may not be an easy matter for some people to limit their exposure to PAHs and other toxins that may trigger esophageal cancer. Carcinogenic substances in combustion products or diesel pollutants make chimney sweeps and people who work in garages at increased risk for this disease. Farmers and other agricultural workers who work with pesticides are also at risk, as are people exposed to beryllium over the long term.

HOT DRINKS AND ESOPHAGEAL CANCER

It may surprise those who regularly enjoy cups of tea or coffee at scalding temperatures that they are increasing their risk for esophageal cancer. Researchers have demonstrated a link between esophageal cancer and drinks served piping hot, such as yerba maté is in southern Brazil.[10] In fact, the data show that when scorching hot maté is drunk in amounts of more than one liter a day, it may become carcinogenic. It is thought that the maté itself as well as the temperature of the drink may trigger cancer. Drinks or other consumables that irritate esophageal tissues, the mouth, or pharynx can also increase the risk for esophageal cancer.

SUMMARY

Lifestyle choices strongly affect risk for esophageal cancer. Several factors are known to increase the risk for this disease, including excessive alcohol consumption, tobacco smoke, consumption of very hot drinks, eating charred foods, being overweight, inactivity, and a diet low in fruit and vegetables. Studies also indicate that eating salted, fermented, and smoked foods increases the risk for this cancer, likely because of nitrosamines and mycotoxins prevalent in some food preparations.

Environmental and occupational factors also play a role, especially PAH exposure. It follows that people may reduce their risk for this disease by avoiding these risk factors while getting plenty of exercise and increasing the amount of fruit and vegetables in their diets.[2] It is important to note that research shows that only some people within an at-risk group will develop esophageal cancer, even when exposed to environmental carcinogens. This suggests that some people may be more genetically vulnerable to this cancer.

Chapter 7

Gastric Cancer

Gastric cancer, also known as stomach cancer, is the second-most-deadly cancer worldwide. Survival rates tend to be poor for this disease as it can progress dangerously far without producing clear symptoms.

The incidence of this cancer, however, varies with location. The highest-risk countries are in Asia, especially Japan, Korea, and China. Other areas with a raised risk for this cancer include South and Central America—where people face an incidence of more than 10 times that in the United States.

In 2010 more than 21,000 people will learn they have stomach cancer in the United States, while about 10,570 will die from the disease.[6] Less than 30 percent of Americans with gastric cancer will survive five years past diagnosis. However, gastric cancer rates have dropped in the United States and many other developed countries in the last 50 years. This is likely due to improved food-handling hygiene, widespread refrigeration, less consumption of salted and preserved foods, and diets richer in fruit and vegetables.[1]

SYMPTOMS

As gastric cancer usually shows few early signs, most people are not diagnosed with this disease until it has advanced. Symptoms typically include loss of appetite, indigestion, stomach pain or discomfort, a bloated feeling after meals, nausea, and heartburn. With time, people with this cancer may vomit for no apparent reason and have weight loss, jaundice (a yellowing of the skin and the whites of the eyes), pain and fluid buildup in their abdomen, trouble swallowing, and blood in their stool. These symptoms may indicate other health problems, too; a prompt visit to the doctor is recommended for a proper diagnosis.

RISK FACTORS

The main factors linked to stomach cancer risk include tobacco use, a poor diet, excessive alcohol consumption, and chronic infection (chronic gastritis or stomach inflammation) from *Helicobacter pylori* (*H. pylori*) bacteria. There is also evidence that some people may have a genetic vulnerability to this disease; studies of twins show higher than expected concordance rates of stomach cancer among identical twins.[2]

Research has shown that first-degree relatives such as parents, siblings, and children of people with stomach cancer have a higher risk for gastric cancer. Very rare familial cancer syndromes, including hereditary nonpolyposis colorectal cancer, juvenile polyposis, and familial adenomatous polyposis, are passed through families.

This chapter has more discussion of these hereditary diseases below. Other than those with these familial syndromes, people who have gastric polyps (caused by inflammation) have a 20 percent higher risk of developing gastric cancer, particularly if they have many polyps and polyps larger than two centimeters in diameter.

In general, men tend to be more susceptible to gastric cancer than women, likely due to lifestyle factors such as drinking alcohol or smoking. Diagnosis usually occurs between the ages of 40 and 60.

H. pylori Bacteria Infection

Research has shown a high rate of gastric cancer in places where many people are infected with *H. pylori*, a bacteria that thrives in the human stomach.[2] Although this bacterial infection does not cause stomach cancer in most people, those who have a persistent infection have a higher risk. One hypothesis is that infection creates chronic inflammation and an increased production of harmful metabolites such as reactive oxygen species. These metabolites damage gastric cell DNA, which may lead to the development of stomach cancer. It's not known why some people are more vulnerable to gastric cell DNA damage and thus to gastric cancer. Most evidence suggests that smoking, poor eating habits, and alcohol abuse can further the damage done by *H. pylori* bacteria and increase a person's chances for gastric cancer.

Someone with an *H. pylori* infection often has no clear symptoms, but people may experience burning back pain, nausea, weight loss, bloating, and gas (burping in particular). A combination of antibiotics can kill the bacteria.

Genetic Factors

Some research points to gene mutations as factors that raise the risk for stomach cancer, especially damage to genes responsible for drug metabolism pathways.

One such mutation on the *N*-acetyltransferase 1 gene is thought to enhance the DNA-damaging effects of various carcinogens, including those found in tobacco smoke.[3]

Other studies have also shown that people may have an increased risk of stomach cancer if they have genetic mutations in an enzyme known as glutathione *S*-transferase, a key player in detoxifying xenobiotics (unwanted foreign substances in the body). The research also suggests that people with genetic mutations in these important enzymes can worsen their chances for gastric cancer if they smoke or abuse alcohol.[3]

Genetic mutations in stomach immune system proteins meant to handle infections such as *H. pylori* can also increase the risk for stomach cancer. The research on damage or mutations in the interleukin gene cluster (responsible for coding for proinflammatory cytokines) shows these mutations can hinder a response to infection or invasion of foreign material. This means the health of a person's immune response in the stomach can show if this person has a higher risk of stomach cancer complication due to *H. pylori* or gastroesophageal reflux (see below).[7,8]

Familial and Autoimmune Disease

Several diseases make people more likely to develop gastric cancer, including autoimmune gastritis (an inherited disease characterized by pernicious anemia and a lack of hydrochloric acid in the stomach), gastric polyps (tumorlike growths), and gastroesophageal reflux disease. As noted above, reflux disease increases the risk for esophageal and stomach cancers. In some cases, the inflamed esophageal or gastric tissue that develops into gastritis or esophagitis at the gastric-esophageal junction (where the esophagus meets the stomach) can later become cancer. It's thought that the inflamed tissue is more vulnerable to carcinogens and oxygen free radicals.[4]

Other diseases linked to a higher risk of stomach cancer are hereditary non-polyposis colorectal cancer (HNPCC) and familial polyposis coli (FPC), a condition usually tied to an increased risk of colorectal cancer (see chapter 5 for more details).

Diet

It's common knowledge that people who eat plenty of antioxidant-rich fruit and vegetables and avoid salt, smoked foods, tobacco, and excess alcohol have a much lower risk of gastric cancer. Widespread use of refrigeration in the developed world has also made it possible to avoid the potentially harmful effects of fungal contamination in food or unhealthy food-preservation techniques.

Yet some areas have a tradition of foods that may increase risk for cancer, including smoked or salted meat and fish. As discussed in chapter 6, "Esophageal

Cancer," nitroso compounds (including the preservative nitrates and nitrites in smoked meat and fish) can be metabolized in the stomach into carcinogenic nitrosamine products. Frying or barbecuing meat at high temperatures or otherwise charring the meat or fish can also produce carcinogens, in this case heterocyclic amines.[9] Some researchers have looked for a connection between dietary cholesterol (from animal fat) and stomach cancer risk but did not find a significant link.[5] All in all, studies show that meat eaters who have an *H. pylori* bacterial infection are at a higher risk for developing stomach cancer.

SUMMARY

Although stomach cancer causes many deaths around the world, the research shows that most of the risk factors for this disease are preventable. Besides eating well and avoiding unhealthy lifestyle habits such as smoking or excessive drinking, people can also practice good sanitation to avoid catching *H. pylori*. But while frequent hand washing, taking care with food safety, and ensuring a fresh, safe supply of drinking water is a matter of course in the West, attaining these goals are big challenges in the developing world.

Chapter 8

Head and Neck Cancer

The term "head and neck cancer" refers to a wide variety of related diseases that develop in the head or neck area. These include cancers of the mouth, lips, sinuses, throat, larynx, salivary glands, and nasal cavity. As a group, these cancers are the sixth-most-common cause of death by cancer. Cancers of the brain, eye, skin, bones, muscles, and scalp are often not considered part of this group.

Although these cancers account for less than 5 percent of cancers diagnosed in the United States, the disease is responsible for many deaths around the globe. The World Health Organization's International Agency for Research on Cancer estimates that about 667,000 people worldwide were diagnosed with lip, oral cavity, larynx, nasopharynx, and pharynx cancers in 2010.[20] About 375,000 were expected to die from these diseases, the majority of them male (accounting for about three-quarters of the deaths).

Head and neck cancers often start in the squamous (scalelike) cells that cover mucosal surfaces within the mouth, nose, and throat—cavity-like areas often exposed to air and the environment. These types of cancers are therefore referred to as head and neck squamous cell carcinomas (HNSCCs) and describe about 90 percent of cases. Of all the head and neck cancers reported in the literature, about 40 percent is reported in the oral cavity, 25 percent in the larynx, and 15 in the pharynx. Another cancer type of the head and neck is adenocarcinoma, which begins in glandular cells such as salivary glands.

AGE AND ETHNICITY

The research shows these diseases tend to strike older people; they are rarely found in people under age 40. In fact, most people with head and neck cancer are older than age 50. However, when people younger than age 45 develop one of these cancers, their chances for survival tend to be poor, even worse if they happen to be an African American male.[1] The mortality rate for African American men is about twice as high as that for Caucasian men. These differences are not seen in women, who have lower overall incidence and death rates.[16,17]

In general, men are much more prone than women to develop head and neck cancers—males are diagnosed with these illnesses four times as often as females. The gap is narrowing, however, as women are seeing rising rates of head and neck cancers, likely due to changes in drinking and smoking habits.

SYMPTOMS

As cancers of the head and neck vary, so do the symptoms. These may include blocked sinuses or chronic sinus infections that do not respond to treatment; unusual nose bleeds or blood or pain in the mouth; recurrent headaches; chronic neck or throat pain; pain when swallowing; white or red patches on gums, tongue, or lining of the mouth; facial numbness or paralysis; swelling around the chin or jawbone; pain or ringing in the ears; difficulty speaking or breathing; difficulty hearing; and voice hoarseness or changes. Of course, these symptoms may indicate health problems other than head and neck cancer; anyone with these symptoms should have a medical or dental examination.

RISK FACTORS

The variety of head and neck cancers also means different risk factors and genetic traits. People who smoke, for example, are exposing their larynxes to the toxic effects of burning tobacco. Or some workplaces may harbor carcinogens that can contribute to head and neck cancer. For example, exposure to airborne asbestos particles is linked to cancer of the larynx. Workers exposed to sulfuric acid mist also have a higher risk for laryngeal cancer, while inhaling wood or nickel dust is linked to cancers in the paranasal sinuses and nasal cavity. Poor oral hygiene, the consumption of particular preservatives and salted foods, and infection with the Epstein-Barr virus are thought to raise one's risk for nasopharynx cancer.[2]

Key Risk Factors: Tobacco, Alcohol, Ultraviolet Exposure, and HPV

The most significant risk factors for head and neck cancer are alcohol and tobacco—especially combined—whether the tobacco is smoked, chewed, or inhaled as snuff. People who habitually use both alcohol and tobacco significantly increase their risk for this group of diseases. Cancers typically associated with alcohol and tobacco use include oral cavity cancers and pharynx and larynx cancers. Tobacco in particular has a connection to about 85 percent of head and neck cancers.[3]

That said, incidence of head and neck cancers among nonsmokers and non-drinkers is increasing. One possibility is excess exposure to the sun and the harmful effects of ultraviolet radiation, especially to the lip area and oral cavity. From 5 to 30 percent of people diagnosed with head and neck cancer are nonsmokers, whose head and neck tumors are thought to have fewer genetic mutations and other DNA abnormalities than smokers' tumors.[5]

Another risk factor for head and neck cancers is human papillomavirus (HPV) infection, the same group of viruses that promote cervical cancer.[4] This viral infection in the head or neck may be a consequence of oral sex.

Other risk factors suggested by research include the following: A diet lacking in vitamin A is a factor that points to an increased risk for cancer of the larynx. As with esophageal cancer, drinking the South American tealike beverage maté, often served piping hot, is linked to a raised risk of mouth, throat, and larynx cancers. As noted in chapter 6 as a risk factor for esophageal cancer, gastroesophageal reflux disease (in which stomach acid backs up into the esophagus) also puts people at a higher risk for head and neck cancers. Irritation of the esophageal lining by the acid reflux (which is therefore associated with esophageal cancer) may extend to the lining of the hypopharynx and can increase the risk for cancer in this location too.

Genetic Factors

Although alcohol and tobacco are strong links for the majority of people who have head and neck cancer, it is still true that most people who drink or smoke, or do both, do not develop these cancers.

Because of this, scientists know other factors are involved in the development of these diseases. Research has shown that some people have particular areas on the structure of their DNA that are more vulnerable to damage, possibly making these people more likely to develop cancer—especially if they are exposed to carcinogens such as those found in cigarette smoke.[18]

Other research suggests that some areas of DNA structure may be fragile in some people, because of inadequate or defective DNA repair mechanisms, and therefore may not be able to contend with the harm done by carcinogens.[19] This research addresses the fact that people with head and neck cancers and defective DNA repair mechanisms tend to have more genetic abnormalities than people with adequate DNA repair mechanisms who have been exposed to similar carcinogens. Scientists have identified more than 150 human DNA repair genes with several distinct DNA repair pathways. Damage to these repair mechanisms are linked to higher risk of cancer, particularly along one known as the base-excision repair (BER) pathway. This pathway is thought to manage a sizable percentage of cytotoxic and mutagenic-induced DNA damage repair and so is of key importance. For example, the DNA damage thought to be done by tobacco smoke can be handled through the BER pathway—but if a person's BER repair mechanism is faulty, this person may be more susceptible to head and neck cancer, especially if he or she is also a smoker.

Several recent studies have shown that mutations in *BER* genes may promote head and neck cancer susceptibility.[4]

Environmental risk factors can compound the problems posed by genetic mutations and promote cancer development. As several genes are involved in the BER process to help the cell deal with various types of DNA injury, germ-line mutations in these essential repair genes may also lead to a higher risk of head and neck cancers.[6,7]

As noted for other types of cancer, damage or mutation in the key regulatory protein p53 has been connected to higher rates of head and neck cancers. The *p53* tumor suppressor gene aids genomic stability by preventing cells from dividing before they are repaired or destroyed (if necessary). Scientists have found mutations that turn off the *p53* tumor suppressor function in at least half of tumors studied, indicating that this gene plays a key role in helping prevent cancer.[8]

Diet and Risk

While studies have shown that people who eat plenty of fruit and vegetables have a lower risk of head and neck cancers, it is not clear what is responsible for these foods' protective qualities. Some theories point to the flavonoids contained in plant foods, shown to have antioxidant properties and other beneficial qualities that may prevent genetic mutations, particularly in respiratory and digestive tract cancers.

Most protective effects have been linked with fruit, although some studies have indicated that eating certain vegetables lowers the risk for head and neck cancers. Studies have also indicated an inverse relationship between eating flavonoid-loaded foods and cancers of the mouth and pharynx—results that were seen to be consistent despite gender, age, education, body mass index, or smoking and drinking habits.[9] (Additional information about the benefits and controversy of food supplements is covered in chapter 21.)

Tobacco

Anyone who has read the preceding chapters will have noticed a pattern: tobacco smoke is the single most important preventable risk factor linked to most cancers, and head and neck cancers are no exception. The reason is that more than 4,000 compounds have been found in tobacco products and so far 63 of them have been found to be carcinogenic, at least 11 of them known to be carcinogenic to people.

The most dangerous among these human carcinogens are polycyclic aromatic hydrocarbons (PAHs) and tobacco-specific nitrosamines and aromatic amines. These toxins harm cell DNA. Research has shown tobacco-related carcinogens such as PAHs in DNA adducts (areas where carcinogens have bonded to DNA, potentially damaging genetic material) in the head and neck cancer cells of smokers. Some scientists believe that this type of carcinogen-induced damage to DNA plays a key role in PAH-induced cancers such as oral cancer.[10]

Alcohol

Drinking alcohol excessively is also a key risk factor for head and neck cancers, particularly if the drink is beer or hard liquor. There does not appear to be a strong link between wine consumption and these types of cancers. This may reflect how wine is consumed, such as with meals; or the effects from wine's components; or the differences between populations and their alcohol preferences.[11,12] It is not clear exactly how drinking excessive amounts of alcohol contributes to head and neck cancer, although a metabolite of the ethanol in alcohol is acetaldehyde, a carcinogen. Unchecked, this toxin can impede DNA function and repair, possibly leading to tumor growth.

The body metabolizes alcohol in steps, the first via an enzyme called alcohol dehydrogenase (ADH2). This process produces acetaldehyde, which is then metabolized by the aldehyde dehydrogenase (ALDH2) enzyme. But these key enzymes can have mutations that have an effect on their function and thus a person's acetaldehyde levels—making them more vulnerable to head and neck cancers.

Aside from metabolic processes, alcoholic drinks may contain carcinogens (carcinogenic activating agents) and contaminants or unidentified harmful compounds, thereby increasing drinkers' risk for head and neck cancer. Or alcoholic drinks may impede the absorption of nutrients, promote carcinogen access within the mouth, depress immune function, and prevent the detoxification of carcinogens.[13]

Infection and Head and Neck Cancers

Scientists are looking closely at connections between chronic infection and inflammation with head and neck cancers. HPV type 16 (HPV16), the virus most strongly linked to cervical cancer, is thought to play a role in these diseases, especially for nonsmokers. The most commonly seen cancers with an HPV connection are squamous cell carcinomas of the tonsils, oropharynx (area of the throat at the back of the mouth), and larynx.

While the immune system conquers most viral infections, some people may have a genetic weakness that predisposes them for infection and, possibly, cancer.[14]

Research has shown that after HPV invades a person's healthy cells, the virus impedes the key tumor suppressor genes known as *p53* and *Rb*. While these human genes normally work to slow cell division to allow repair or elimination of damaged cells, these functions are overthrown after HPV enters the cell and inserts its own genes to be duplicated courtesy of the human cell. Other viruses found in head and neck cancers—suggesting a causal link—include the Epstein-Barr virus, human herpesvirus type 8, and bovine leukemia.

Bacteria thought to cause periodontitis, a chronic oral infection also known as gum disease, may also increase risk for head and neck cancer when acting alongside viral infections such as HPV, the Epstein-Barr virus, and cytomegalovirus. Studies indicate that viruses may find safe haven in periodontal pockets. Periodontitis creates a chronic release of substances linked to cancer development including enzymes, chemokines, prostaglandins, growth factors, and inflammatory cytokines. Significant evidence links chronic infections with a higher risk of head and neck cancer.[15]

SUMMARY

The exact causes of head and neck cancer are unknown, although the most significant risk factors can be avoided with lifestyle adjustments. These risk factors include tobacco smoke, chronic alcohol abuse, and HPV infection—all risk factors for other types of cancer as well.

Chapter 9

Leukemia and Lymphoma

Leukemia is one of the more rare cancers, accounting for about 3 percent of all new cancer cases in the United States. About 43,000 people are diagnosed with leukemia in this country annually, with about half that many dying every year, according to the National Cancer Institute.[22] Although rare, this disease is the most common type of cancer in children, amounting to 30 percent of cancers in people younger than age 15.[1]

In a nutshell, leukemia is a cancer of the blood's white cells, the cells that play a prime defense role in the body's immune system. Cancer in these cells is unlike other types of cancer, which develop in solid tissue. As white blood cells are created in the bone marrow, so is this type of cancer, which then moves into the blood and flows to areas throughout the body. This is why leukemia tumors are referred to as liquid tumors.

We've also included discussion on lymphoma cancers, which form in immune system cells instead of bone marrow and so are not considered leukemia. Multiple myeloma, on the other hand, is a rare type of cancer that some deem a type of leukemia.

TYPES OF LEUKEMIA

There are two main types of leukemia: myeloid leukemia (also called nonlymphocytic leukemia) and lymphoid leukemia (or lymphocytic leukemia).

Myeloid Leukemia

Myeloid leukemia originates in young myeloid cells, such as nonlymphocyte white blood cells, red blood cells, or platelet-making cells. When cancer develops, immature forms of these cells have accumulated without achieving the ability to fight disease or infection.

Lymphocytic Leukemia

Lymphocytic (lymphoid) leukemia first develops in the immature white blood cells, or lymphocytes, that are part of the body's defense system to fight infections. Usually, white blood cells called lymphocytes are made and die off systematically. But when leukemia develops in bone marrow (where the cells are made), abnormal cells accumulate and impede normal defense functions.

Both types of leukemia can in turn be considered chronic or acute. In acute leukemia, the disease develops quickly as abnormal and immature blood cells multiply rapidly. Chronic leukemia may show fewer symptoms in its early stages, and it advances more slowly. Acute lymphocytic leukemia (ALL) is the most common leukemia in US children and can be treated successfully. Chronic leukemia in either form is not commonly found among children but is often seen in adults with leukemia and acute myeloid leukemia (AML).

Symptoms and Treatment

Leukemia cells travel through the body, so symptoms depend on the location and number of gathered cells. Some people with chronic leukemia will not experience symptoms, but others with chronic or acute leukemia may have swollen lymph nodes (usually pain free), fatigue and weakness, weight loss, fevers or night sweats, joint pain, and headaches or seizures (if leukemia has traveled to the brain). A variety of treatments are used for leukemia patients, including chemotherapy, radiation, and stem cell transplantation. Even if a patient's symptoms disappear, therapy may be needed to prevent a relapse.

PROBABLE CAUSES

Research has linked several risk factors to leukemia, although the connections are not well understood. One of leukemia's most obvious possible causes includes high levels of radiation exposure, such as from the atomic bomb explosions during World War II in Japan or from the Chernobyl nuclear power plant accident in 1986. Another type of high-level exposure comes from medical radiation treatments; in contrast, medical devices used for diagnosis involve lower radiation levels and are not associated with cancer.[2]

Environmental toxins may contribute to risk, such as cigarette smoke or workplace exposure to pesticides, herbicides and harsh solvents.[3] Some occupations may offer particular risks. For example, workers in the rubber, petrochemical, and pharmaceutical industries may be exposed to benzene, a highly flammable liquid connected to a higher risk of leukemia.[4] Another high-risk substance used in chemical plants is formaldehyde.

Some people may be genetically more susceptible to leukemia; several familial conditions can increase family members' risk. Studies have revealed some DNA or chromosomal abnormalities in leukemia patients' blood cells. Patients with Down syndrome, for example, have chromosomal abnormalities along with a higher risk for leukemia.[5]

Viral infections, diseases, and other conditions that disrupt immune function may also play a role in the development of leukemia. For instance, the human T-cell leukemia virus (HTLV-I) causes human T-cell leukemia, an unusual form of chronic lymphocytic leukemia. The blood disease myelodysplastic syndrome, a stem cell disorder that harms a person's ability to create normal cells, increases patients' risk for acute myeloid leukemia. Although it remains controversial, only a weak association has linked electromagnetic fields from power lines (or other low-energy radiation exposure) to leukemia in children, while no link so far has been found for the disease in adults (see chapter 20 for more discussion on this issue).

RISK FACTORS FOR MYELOID LEUKEMIA

Ionizing Radiation

The connection between leukemia and large doses of ionizing radiation has been known for some time, due to the increased rates of acute and chronic forms of myeloid leukemia in Japanese atomic bomb survivors. Following the Chernobyl accident in 1986, children born to radiation-exposed parents experienced high rates of leukemia.[15] Workplace research has also shown higher rates for acute myeloid leukemia in people who work in the nuclear industry (rates remain higher even today because of the higher risk of radiation and benzene exposure) and for more leukemia deaths than expected for radiologists in the science's early days.[16]

Several factors are thought to affect how radiation exposure promotes leukemia: the dose, the type of exposure, the age of the person at exposure, and the time lapse since the exposure. The radiation damages DNA, possibly through ionization or by producing harmful reactive free radicals that disrupt DNA. As a result, necessary genes in the affected cells cannot perform key functions and cancer develops.

A single dose of high radiation or several installments of fractionated radiotherapy (dose of radiation divided over a number of treatments) increases a person's risk for chronic and acute myeloid leukemia and for acute lymphocytic leukemia.

Tobacco Smoke

Leukemia is yet another cancer linked to cigarette smoke. Some reports show an association between smoking and adult leukemia, especially acute myeloid leukemia. The data are not consistent regarding tobacco smoke and leukemia in children, however. For example, results from case-control studies on paternal and maternal smoking and the risk of acute lymphocytic leukemia and acute myeloid leukemia in children did not show an increased risk for these cancers due to maternal smoking alone, possibly because women may smoke fewer tobacco cigarettes during their pregnancies. Conversely, fathers' pre-conception smoking showed a significant increase in the risk for these cancers.[6]

Interestingly, the researchers noted the highest risk for acute lymphocytic leukemia was for a combination of fathers' pre-conception smoking with mothers' postnatal smoking or their postnatal passive tobacco smoke exposure. This is compared to fathers' pre-conception smoking alone.

Some research offers explanations of why paternal pre-conception smoking may pose a leukemia risk for unborn children. One team found 50 percent higher levels of a product of oxidative DNA damage (8-hydroxy-2'-deoxyguanosine) in smokers' sperm compared to nonsmokers' sperm.[8]

Other studies have also linked smoking to oxidative damage and aneuploidy (abnormal chromosome copy number) in the sperm of smokers. Whether they were light or heavy smokers, tobacco users were found to be much more likely to produce abnormal sperm than nonsmokers. Smoking mothers, meanwhile, increase the risk of chromosomal damage in their newborns.[6]

As tobacco smoke is rife with carcinogens, it is perhaps not surprising that it is linked with childhood leukemia. At least 63 of the more than 4,000 compounds in this smoke are carcinogenic, with 11 of them known to cause cancer in people. These poisons include polycyclic aromatic hydrocarbons (PAHs) and tobacco-specific nitrosamines (TSNs) that harm cell DNA.

Some studies have examined toxin levels in children after cigarette smoke exposure. One study found high levels of DNA-damaging serum cotinine (a chemical the body produces from nicotine), 4-aminobiphenyl-hemoglobin adduct, and PAH-albumin adducts. The children studied were exposed daily to the smoke of about 10½ cigarettes from their mothers and about 6½ from visitors. The compounds found in the children are linked not only to leukemia but to other cancers.[7]

Benzene

Research has shown a strong connection between benzene exposure and leukemia, especially for myeloid leukemia. Myeloid progenitor cells are more susceptible to harm from benzene than mature white blood cells, thus myeloid cancers are more common with this type of exposure.

Even low-level exposures of this toxin in the workplace can cause higher levels of cancer-associated DNA abnormalities. In addition, workers who smoke are more at risk for leukemia when exposed to benzene, as cigarette smoke already contains benzene. The average smoker is exposed to 2 milligrams of benzene daily, with about 90 percent of the dose coming from cigarettes. In contrast, non-smokers are usually exposed to about 0.2 milligrams of benzene daily, typically from outdoor air, indoor air, automobiles, and passive smoke.[6]

Familial Syndromes

Some people inherit conditions that make them more likely to develop leukemia. They may have a family history of a blood clotting problem (familial platelet disorder), abnormal production of red blood cells (sideroblastic anemia), or diseases such as neurofibromatosis type 1 or polyposis coli.

Other hereditary diseases that increase the risk for leukemia are congenital immunodeficiency disorders, Li-Fraumeni syndrome (a hereditary disorder that increases susceptibility to cancer), pediatric acute lymphocytic leukemia, and Bloom syndrome (a chromosomal disorder). Furthermore, a person's risk for leukemia rises when family members have other cancers such as breast cancer. In these rare families, the extra risk is often due to inheritable mutations in a key tumor suppressor gene, *p53*.[9]

Genetic Syndromes

In simple terms, leukemia is caused by direct or indirect damage to myeloid or lymphoblastic cells. When cells' repair mechanisms are harmed, they can no longer fix or otherwise manage injured DNA. This kind of damage has a significant association with the promotion and progression of leukemia (and lymphoma). Families with enzyme mutations that impede DNA mismatch repairs (or otherwise prove to be genetically unstable) likely have more genetic abnormalities and, consequently, a higher risk for early-onset leukemia. Studies of leukemia cells have found frequent chromosomal translocations (a chromosomal abnormality due to chromosomal breaks that rejoin to other chromosomes), often resulting in unbalanced translocations and the loss of chromosomal material.

Children with Down syndrome have an increased risk of leukemia, possibly because of the chromosomal abnormality that causes their condition. The major chromosomal irregularity among children with Down syndrome is having three copies of chromosome 21, instead of the normal two chromosomes. Chromosome 21 is often involved in acute lymphocytic leukemia and acute myeloid leukemia in people with this chromosomal disorder. The disease process that leads to childhood leukemia in children with Down syndrome can start early—often in utero.[6]

LYMPHOMA CANCERS

Lymphomas begin in the cells and tissues of the body's lymphatic system, part of the body's immune system. The lymphatic system includes the lymph nodes (clusters of white blood cells) and other lymphatic tissues. Lymphomas develop when malformed lymphocytes proliferate, overwhelming and hindering the normal function of the lymph nodes. Worse, these cancerous cells can travel throughout the body to various organs or the bone marrow by virtue of the lymphatic system's wide reach. About 5 percent of Americans with cancer have lymphomas.

The two types of lymphomas are Hodgkin lymphoma (or Hodgkin disease) and non-Hodgkin lymphoma, each quite different in how the body is affected and how the cancer responds to treatment.

Both Hodgkin and Non-Hodgkin lymphoma originate in the lymphatic cells. The main difference between the two types of cancer is that Hodgkin lymphoma is associated with abnormal cells called Reed-Sternberg cells, whereas Non-Hodgkin lymphoma is associated with the absence of Reed-Sternberg cells.

Hodgkin Lymphoma

A rare type of lymphoma, Hodgkin lymphoma tends to occur more often in males and in people from a higher socioeconomic sphere. People with parents or siblings with this disease have a higher risk, especially if the ill family member is younger than age 40. About 8,480 new cases of Hodgkin lymphoma were expected in the United States in 2010 and an estimated 1,320 deaths from the disease, according to the National Cancer Institute.[23]

Symptoms and Treatment

Typical symptoms for this disease include the painless swelling of lymph nodes, spleen, or other immune tissue; fever; tiredness; night sweats; and weight loss. The good news is that many patients with Hodgkin lymphoma can have their disease managed for years or even be cured, thanks to recent scientific advances.

Non-Hodgkin Lymphoma

More than 20 malignant diseases are included in this group, all springing from T and B lymphocytes (white blood cells); 70 to 80 percent of them grow in lymph nodes.

This cancer is rare in children; most new cases of this disease are in men older than age 70. Non-Hodgkin lymphoma is the sixth-most-common cancer in men, following lung, colon, prostate, bladder, and melanoma. However, it is the fifth-most-common cancer in women, following lung, breast, colon, and melanoma, and the third-most-common cancer in children younger than 14. About 65,540 new cases of non-Hodgkin lymphoma were expected in the United States in 2010; about 20,210 Americans died from the disease that year, according to the National Cancer Institute.[24]

Symptoms and Treatment

Symptoms for this disease include enlarged lymph nodes, weight loss, and fever; the stage and type of cancer determine the prognosis, as well as the person's age and overall health. Treatment options may include chemotherapy, radiation therapy, targeted therapy, or participation in clinical trials of new treatments such as vaccine therapy (intended to assist patients' immune systems in fighting cancer), or high-dose chemotherapy with stem cell implant. Some doctors may also advise a wait-and-see approach, meaning no treatment until symptoms change.

Lymphoma Risk Factors

Commonly associated risk factors for lymphoma cancers include autoimmune diseases that hinder the immune system, such as HIV-AIDS; viral infections such as the Epstein-Barr virus; genetic mutations that promote abnormal cell growth; immunosuppressive therapeutic drug treatment; and bacteria-induced gastric disease.

HIV-AIDS and Lymphoma

Scientific research shows that people infected with the human immunodeficiency virus (HIV) have a significantly higher risk of non-Hodgkin lymphoma. Among other effects, HIV creates a chronic stimulation of B cells; about 90 percent of non-Hodgkin lymphoma cases in people with HIV are linked to the proliferation of these cells.[10]

Epstein-Barr Virus

About 90 percent of adults around the world have been infected with the Epstein-Barr virus (EBV). A herpesvirus, it typically infects people in their early years, with a latent infection enduring all their lives. While some people may not experience much harm from this infection, cells infected with EBV have a growth advantage and may not die the way healthy cells eventually do (this effect is a bit like cancer's effects on cells). Normally, the immune system uses its cells to quickly eliminate pathogens, but EBV-infected immune cells are no longer functional this way. As the immune system is the body's first defense against pathogens—including cancer cells—a person's defense systems are weakened when flooded with EBV. This can leave the system vulnerable to cancer.

Solid evidence shows that people with weak immune systems, such as during a post-transplant period or after HIV-AIDS infection, have an increased risk of non-Hodgkin lymphoma if they are also infected with the Epstein-Barr virus. In Africa, this ubiquitous virus is also linked to Burkett lymphoma in children.[11]

Autoimmune Diseases

Autoimmune diseases, such as lupus or rheumatoid arthritis, occur when the immune system fails to recognize itself and launches its defenses, resulting in inflammatory disease. It is not yet fully understood why, but there is a positive association between non-Hodgkin lymphoma and autoimmune diseases. Most of the research on this topic has been through cohort studies of small groups with autoimmune disease, not case-control studies of non-Hodgkin lymphoma risk.

And most of the data for the non-Hodgkin lymphoma connection with autoimmune disease are concerned with rheumatoid arthritis. This helps fuel the debate on whether the increased cancer risk is because of the autoimmune disease itself or because of treatment with immune-suppressive drugs (such as steroids or azathioprine).

Although less data are available, researchers have linked several other autoimmune diseases with a moderately higher risk of this cancer. These include systemic lupus erythema, Sjorgren syndrome, psoriasis, and celiac disease. People with allergic and atopic conditions, however, are thought to have a lower risk of non-Hodgkin lymphoma.[12]

Familial Lymphoma

People with a family history of malignant lymphomas also appear to have a higher risk for lymphoma, especially if the family incidence of cancer is located in tissue where new blood cells are formed (hematopoietic tissue). The family link suggests that hereditary or genetic factors may be important in the development of these cancers. Some reports indicate that first-degree relatives of people with non-Hodgkin lymphoma face twice the risk of developing the cancer themselves. The risk of Hodgkin lymphoma to first-degree relatives of patients with this cancer is thought to be even higher.

Studies investigating risk for non-Hodgkin lymphoma for people with or without familial hematopoietic cancer found that familial hematopoietic cancer increases the non-Hodgkin lymphoma risk when combined with a variety of behaviors and exposures. The research included homosexual behavior, drug use, pesticide exposure, occupational contaminant exposure, history of liver disease, and alcohol consumption—all more strongly linked to an increased cancer risk for men with a family history of hematopoietic cancer. The data suggest a combination of nongenetic and genetic risk factors may affect lymphoma risk.[13]

Post-transplant Immunosuppression and Lymphoma

Immunosuppressive drugs taken to stop the body from rejecting transplanted organs or tissues appear to increase the transplant patient's risk for non-Hodgkin lymphoma. Reports show that 22 percent of all people who developed cancer after receiving a transplant developed non-Hodgkin lymphoma (the results exclude those with nonmelanoma skin cancer). This risk drops significantly one year after the transplant operation.

Pesticides, Herbicides, and Agricultural Exposures

Some research has focused on the risks of non-Hodgkin lymphoma to those involved in the manufacturing or use of herbicides and pesticides. These studies found a link between this cancer and exposure to PCBs (polychlorinated biphenyls) but not to DDT (dichlorodiphenyltrichloroethane) or related pesticides. While it appears that farmers have a slightly higher risk of non-Hodgkin lymphoma, it is not yet known why. The list for potential risk factors related to non-Hodgkin lymphoma in farming is long: pesticides, herbicides, fungicides, infectious microorganisms, paints, oils, solvents, fuels, and dust.[17]

More research is needed to determine what exposures or lifestyle habits particular to farmers can explain their higher risk for non-Hodgkin lymphoma.

Multiple Myeloma

Amounting to about 1 percent of all cancers, multiple myeloma is a very rare type of blood cancer that differs from leukemia and lymphoma in that it occurs in mature blood plasma cells. Multiple myeloma can then grow without limits, hindering blood production and commonly causing anemia as an early symptom. About 40 percent of patients with multiple myeloma develop plasma cell leukemia.[18] This disease could be considered a type of leukemia, although derived from plasma cells. Some researchers hypothesize that multiple myeloma and leukemia coexist.[19]

Patients with this disease are typically older; men develop this cancer one and a half times as often as women, and African Americans have double the risk of Caucasians. African Americans tend to develop this disease at a younger age; the median age for African Americans is age 67 at diagnosis, for Caucasians it is age 71.[20,21]

Symptoms

The usual symptoms include infections, neurological deficits (a decrease in brain, spinal cord, muscle, or nerve activity), renal failure, hypercalcemia, and bone or rib pain.

Risk Factors for Multiple Myeloma

Research results indicate that first-degree relatives of people with multiple myeloma are at a higher risk for the disease. The risk appears to be increased yet again for people whose relatives had late-onset multiple myeloma, especially for women although it is not known why. Neither is much known about the risk factors for this rare cancer. However, case-control and cohort studies have suggested that radiologists exposed to ionizing radiation (after long latency periods) and some farmers and petrochemical and rubber industry workers are at higher risk for this disease.[14]

SUMMARY

The direct causes of leukemia and other diseases discussed in this chapter are not well understood. However, the available evidence points to several factors that can increase risk for disease, particularly for leukemia. These include exposure to ionizing radiation, benzene, pesticides, herbicides, viral and bacterial infections, and tobacco smoke.

On that note, it's public knowledge that women who smoke when they are pregnant risk their children's health in a variety of ways, including increasing their risk for leukemia. But studies have shown that fathers also raise their children's risk for this cancer if they smoke even before their children are conceived, as well as afterward. The research suggests that the timing and sequence of tobacco smoke exposure, passive or otherwise, may be important in the development of childhood leukemia.

As with other cancers, most people who have known risk factors do not develop leukemia, and many people with these types of cancers have none of these risk factors.

Chapter 10

Liver Cancer

Also known as hepatocellular carcinoma, liver cancer is the fifth-most-common cancer in men, and the seventh-most-common cancer in women, globally.[15] Nearly 85 percent of the cases occur in developing nations. Liver cancer's mortality rate is close to its incidence rate: about 788,000 people around the world developed liver cancer in 2010, and roughly 730,000 died from the disease, according to the International Agency for Research on Cancer.[16] In the United States, the National Cancer Institute estimates that 24,000 new cases of liver cancer appeared in 2010, while about 19,000 people died from the disease that year.[17]

The prognosis is poor for those diagnosed with this cancer, although for some the outlook is especially pessimistic. In the West, less than 5 percent survive past five years; in developing countries the survival rate is worse. People in developing countries also become ill with liver cancer as young adults or even as children, while in the West, most people with this disease are over age 60.

Researchers believe that early childhood exposure to this cancer's risk factors may play a significant role in and increase the risk for liver cancer in some parts of the world. One clue is the prevalence of hepatitis B virus infection and aflatoxin (naturally occurring mycotoxins produced by a species of fungus) exposure, both thought to be liver cancer risk factors in Southeast Asia and sub-Saharan Africa, areas with high liver cancer incidence.

In fact, chronic hepatitis B virus infection can begin before age five, even in utero via the placenta. Other risk factors linked to liver cancer include natural and synthetic chemical carcinogens, the use of steroid hormones, the liver damage from diabetes, and cirrhosis as a result of fatty liver disease. Levels of obesity and diabetes continue to rise in the United States and other countries around the world, making this last point significant to many.[1] Men are twice as likely as women to develop liver cancer, possibly because of lifestyle choices such as smoking or drinking excess alcohol or putting themselves more at risk for hepatitis B virus infection (through drug use, for example). People with close relations with this disease may also be more at risk. Of course, cancer is a risk for liver cancer: cells from cancers in other parts of the body can spread to the liver.

Symptoms and Treatment

Liver cancer tends not to produce symptoms until it has advanced. These symptoms include bloating, weight loss, low appetite, fullness, fatigue, nausea, vomiting, dark urine, jaundice, and pain in the upper right area of the abdomen and the back and shoulder. These symptoms are not sure signs of liver cancer and may be caused by other diseases and conditions. Anyone experiencing these symptoms should see a doctor promptly. Treatment options may involve surgery, chemotherapy, radiation therapy, immunotherapy, and vaccine therapy.

RISK FACTORS

Hepatitis B or C Infection

Infections with the hepatitis B virus (HBV) or hepatitis C virus (HCV) are top risk factors for liver cancer. This is because these diseases can cause the chronic inflammation that may ultimately lead to the disease.[2] But while these two viruses may seem alike, they belong to separate viral families and are genetically dissimilar. In fact, HVC infection creates less of a risk for liver cancer than HBV infection.

HBV infection in particular is thought to be carried by more than 400 million people in developing world, where chronic infection in high-HBV-risk countries is estimated to account for up to 94 percent of liver cancer cases. In these areas where HBV is prevalent, this virus is blamed for close to 100 percent of liver cancers in children. In low-risk countries, HBV infection causes up to 10 percent of all cases of liver cancer.[12]

Both viruses can be caught through blood transfusions, through the sharing of needles (such as those for drug use, tattooing, or body piercing), or through sexual activity. Infected mothers can pass these viruses to their babies.

Of course, not everyone who catches one of these viruses develops the same illness; some will be healthy carriers and others will develop acute or chronic hepatitis, liver cirrhosis, or even liver cancer.

How these viruses work in the body is by the HCV or HBV acting on liver cell proteins by inserting their genes into healthy cells. The virus's genetic material then usurps the host cell's genes, forcing the host cell to produce the proteins needed to make more viruses. Now the cell can no longer perform its duties correctly. Worse, HBV binds to the key tumor suppressor gene, $p53$, which helps stop cancer by slowing down cell division so that damaged DNA can be repaired. When $p53$ is damaged or mutated, it cannot stop cells from dividing with defective DNA.

Although HBV is considered the "second-most-important human carcinogen" so far discovered (after tobacco), a chronic infection does not necessarily mean that liver cancer will develop.[12]

Dietary Aflatoxin Exposure

Produced by the *Aspergillus flavus* mold, aflatoxin is a carcinogen found on some types of grains, nuts, or peanuts that have been poorly stored.[6] It is currently the only exogenous mutagen (external agents that cause mutations) in food demonstrated to increase the risk of liver cancer in people. It is also known to boost the cancer-promoting effects of viral hepatitis, a risk especially for people in sub-Saharan Africa and Asia, both places where rates of hepatitis infection are high.

The dangers of aflatoxin B1 first came to light in 1959 in Great Britain when the toxin was found in moldy animal feed after an outbreak of an animal illness known as Turkey X disease.[4] It is now known that while animals that ingest high levels of this poison will likely die, even consuming nontoxic amounts has been shown to lead to liver cancer in animals.

While preventing HBV infection and chronic aflatoxin exposure would greatly reduce the rates of liver cancer in some parts of the world, unfortunately, exposure to both of these carcinogens tends to happen early in life. Research in western Africa has shown that aflatoxin exposure may begin in utero and persist throughout childhood and later adult life. This long-term carcinogen exposure allows for the buildup of DNA damage that can lead to liver cancer.

Geography may be important when looking at aflatoxin as a risk for liver cancer. While this carcinogen poses a significant risk in Africa and Asia, considering the high rates of HBV infection in those areas, in Europe and North America the bigger risk factors for liver cancer may be tobacco smoke and excess alcohol consumption.

HBV Infection, Aflatoxin Exposure Increase Cancer Risk

Epidemiological and animal studies show that the combination of HBV infection and aflatoxin exposure increases the risk for liver cancer, although the mechanisms for this process are not well understood.[7] Research with laboratory mice genetically engineered to mimic human HBV carriers suggests that chronic liver injury (such as that done by HBV) may prevent key enzymes from removing carcinogens, including aflatoxin, from cells. Thus, aflatoxin's harmful effects on DNA continue in the liver, setting the stage for disease.

Cirrhosis

Several types of infections and substance abuses can harm liver tissue and cause scarring in a condition called cirrhosis. A cirrhotic liver loses function and becomes more diseased as scar tissue replaces healthy tissue, preventing blood circulation throughout this essential organ. But the liver cancer risk linked to cirrhosis is not especially high; reports suggest that only about 5 percent of cirrhosis patients develop liver cancer.

The liver cancer–cirrhosis link seems to depend on relevant risk factors. Persistent HBV and HBC infections, chronic alcoholism, tobacco smoke, and a variety of drugs and chemicals are thought to increase the risk for liver cirrhosis. Some research demonstrated that people with two or more of those infections or behaviors are also increasing their risk for liver cancer. For example, a person who chronically drinks excess alcohol and who has an HCV infection has a significantly higher liver cancer risk than most alcoholics with cirrhosis of the liver but no HCV infection or other risk factors.[3]

Chronic Inflammation

Research suggests that chronic inflammation may be a risk factor for many cancers, including liver cancer. This risk appears to depend on genetic mutations or altered gene expression in key players in the body's immune response called cytokines. For example, scientists found mutations in proinflammatory Th1 and anti-inflammatory Th2 cytokines in cancerous liver tissue samples but not in healthy liver tissue samples.[5]

Heavy, Long-Term Alcohol Use and Cigarette Smoke

While people who chronically drink excessive amounts of alcohol have a higher risk for liver cancer, those who drink moderately (one to three alcoholic beverages per day) do not have a higher risk for this disease. Because alcohol is metabolized in the liver, the risk linked to alcohol consumption appears to depend on liver exposure to one of the initial metabolites of alcohol, acetyladehyde, a known carcinogen. Scientists believe that the longer the liver is exposed to acetyladehyde, the more likely it is that liver cells will be harmed. Thus the more alcohol consumed, the more acetyladehyde must be processed in the liver—increasing the toxic effects of this metabolite.

Some people have genetic mutations in the enzymes needed to convert alcohol into acetyladehyde (alcohol dehydrogenase, or ADH2) or break down acetaldehyde (aldehyde dehydrogenase, or ALDH2). These mutations can have a great impact on a person's blood acetaldehyde concentrations after consuming alcohol.

While rare in European populations, these mutations are common to people in China, Korea, Thailand, and Japan. For them, drinking alcohol can greatly increase the risk for liver cancer as the mutations increase their serum acetaldehyde levels to 13 times as high as that of someone without the mutations. This defective alcohol metabolizing mechanism also increases the risk for esophageal cancer. Typically, after drinking alcohol, a person with these mutations will experience a reddened face, nausea, sleepiness, and headache.

As will be discussed further in the next chapter on lung cancer, tobacco smoke is a key risk factor for several cancers, including liver cancer. This complex, toxic smog contains at least 11 known human carcinogens among its more than 4,000 compounds. Its polycyclic aromatic hydrocarbons and tobacco-specific nitrosamines alone have been shown to promote liver cancer in animals. A properly functioning liver clears out toxins, carcinogens, and other chemical agents from the body. But researchers believe long-term exposure to harmful tobacco smoke metabolites may overwhelm healthy liver function, leaving liver cells at risk for cancer. And adding chronic alcoholism to the stress of tobacco smoke on an already overworked liver may dramatically increase one's risk for liver cancer.

Genetic Factors

The research indicates that some people have genetic abnormalities that may make them more susceptible to liver cancer, particularly if they also have other risk factors such as HBV or HCV infections and aflatoxin exposure.

Scientists found significantly more mutated $p53$ tumor suppressor genes in liver cancer tissue samples than in healthy liver tissue samples. A mutated tumor suppressor gene may not be able function properly to stop cells with DNA damage for repair or removal before replication.[8,9] In addition, $p53$ mutation have been linked to the oxidative DNA damage that occurs in the development of liver cancer.

The transforming growth factor (TGF) signaling pathway (a cellular system governing cell growth, cell differentiation, and programmed cell death) is key for healthy cellular activities. In the liver, the TGF pathway keeps in check the regeneration of hepatocytes (cells from main liver tissues) by preventing DNA synthesis and inducing cell death when necessary. However, studies show that in liver cancer, the TGF pathway is overexpressed, possibly leading to a higher rate of tumor angiogenesis (the growth of new blood vessels that pushes benign tumors closer to becoming malignant).

Studies on liver cancer tissue also show other mutated genes with diverse functions that no longer may be performed accurately. It is possible that these other mutated genes also promote liver cancer. The good news is that one day it may be possible to identify and use these genetic mutations as a way to screen for early liver cancer.

PREVENTION

Coffee Drinking and Risk of Liver Cancer

Millions may be pleased to know that their coffee habit may contribute to a reduced risk of liver cancer. Studies, including on animals, suggest that those who enjoy a cup of coffee every day or near daily have a lower risk for liver cancer than those who rarely sip a cup. The liver cancer risk appears to have an inverse relationship with the amount of coffee sipped.

Why this is so continues to be the subject of investigation. Several substances in coffee are of interest, including caffeine and the generous amount of antioxidants, such as chlorogenic acid.

But green tea also contains caffeine and is rich in antioxidant catechins, yet green tea does not have as strong an association with a reduced liver cancer risk. It appears that, as the antioxidant components of these beverages are different, so are the accompanying benefits (see chapter 17, "Nutrition and Cancer," for more information on the benefits found in green tea).

One study found that cup for cup, soluble coffee offers more antioxidants than green tea.[13] It may be that the reduced liver cancer risk seen in coffee drinkers is due to substances yet to be identified in the popular brew. As coffee is sipped in countries around the world, many types of drinking habits have been recorded with intriguing results. For example, epidemiological studies in Brazil of Japanese immigrants documented significant decreases in death from liver disease and cancer, compared with Japanese in Japan, regardless of the high rate of HBV infection in the area. This suggests that factors in the immigrants' new environment may prevent chronic liver disease and liver cancer. As these immigrants moved to coffee-rich Brazil, it is possible that a key factor is the adoption of coffee-drinking habits.[10]

Liver Cancer Vaccine

As a person with a chronic HBV infection is about 100 times more likely to die from liver cancer than a person without the infection, according to one study,[14] a vaccine to prevent HBV infection may make sense. Viral hepatitis alone kills about 1.5 million people annually, although most people who become infected with this virus simply develop an antibody against it and don't get sick.

Research demonstrates that a vaccination program decreases the number of HBV carriers in some communities. Such a vaccine may also prevent deaths from liver cancer, as about 60 percent of liver cancers globally have a connection to hepatitis B.[14] Vaccines are also available for hepatitis A and C. Vaccines must be used on people who are not already infected to protect them against chronic HBV infection and liver cancer.[11]

SUMMARY

Liver cancer causes many illnesses and deaths around the world. Yet several risk factors for this disease are known and preventable. These include tobacco smoke, chronic alcohol consumption, aflatoxin exposure, and hepatitis virus infections—also known to compound the toxic effects of aflatoxin. This suggests that measures to reduce aflatoxin exposure to populations where hepatitis infection (particularly HBV infection) is common would likely reduce the number of people who become ill with liver cancer.

All the same, not everyone exposed to liver cancer's known risk factors will develop the disease, and not all people with liver cancer have been exposed to these risk factors.

Chapter 11

Lung Cancer

It may be the second-most-common type of cancer, but of all the different cancer diseases, lung cancer kills the most men and women. Usually this is because the disease is often discovered at an advanced stage. In 2010 about 222,520 people in the United States were diagnosed with lung cancer, while close to 157,300 died from the disease, according to figures from the National Cancer Institute.[23] Unfortunately, the prognosis is often not encouraging for those with lung cancer. Only about 15.8 percent of patients survive to five years past diagnosis.

The majority of these cancer deaths are caused by tobacco smoke, making this disease the leading cause of avoidable mortality in the United States. In fact, cancers of the lung, bronchus, and trachea are the leading cause of cancer-related deaths in many parts of the world. More on cancer risk and tobacco smoke follows later in this chapter.

Another factor in this disease is age: lung cancer is very rare in anyone younger than 44. Chances for getting this disease increase with age: the median age of diagnosis is 72; most people with this disease are older than age 55.

The good news is that thanks to public health programs, smoking bans, and other lung cancer prevention efforts, lung cancer incidence and mortality rates are dropping in the United States and other Western countries. However, this is not true for some places where tobacco smoking is becoming more popular, such as China and India.

SYMPTOMS AND TREATMENT

Lung cancer usually forms in the cells blanketing the air passages in lung tissues. The disease is classified as one of two main types: small cell lung cancer and non–small cell lung cancer. Most people with lung cancer do not notice any early symptoms. As the disease progresses, they may develop a hoarse voice; a persistent and worsening cough, possibly bringing up blood; trouble breathing; chest pain; chronic lung infections including pneumonia; unexplained weight loss; and extreme fatigue. It's important to note that these symptoms may be caused by health issues other than cancer, although any who have these symptoms should see their doctor promptly.

Doctors may use blood tests, physical examinations, and x-rays and check the sputum for cancer cells or recommend a computed tomography (CT) scan. Treatment is difficult, hence the need for early detection, which improves the chances of successful treatment with surgery, chemotherapy, radiation therapy, and targeted therapy.

Gender, Ethnicity, and Lung Cancer

African Americans have the highest lung cancer incidence and mortality rates of any racial group in the United States. Scientists believe this is because of poor socioeconomic status and unhealthy lifestyle that may include smoking, alcohol abuse, and poor dietary choices. Incidence and mortality is higher in men than in women, mainly due to lifestyle choices, such as smoking.

RISK FACTORS, OTHER THAN TOBACCO

While tobacco smoke is the chief cause in most cases of lung cancer, not everyone who smokes will get lung cancer or any other cancer diseases. Conversely, about 10 percent of people with lung cancer have never smoked. These cases are referred to as "lung cancer cases in never-smokers" (LCINS). A disproportionate amount of these nonsmokers with lung cancer are women. Scientists believe that lung cancer among never-smokers may be caused by inherited genetic susceptibility or by exposure to radon, air pollution, asbestos, cooking fumes, heavy metals, human papillomavirus infection, and environmental tobacco smoke.[4]

People who have had chronic lung diseases such as tuberculosis or bronchitis may also have a higher risk for lung cancer. This is because these diseases can damage the lungs and leave them more susceptible to toxins and the carcinogenic effects that could lead to lung cancer. It's possible a shared genetic susceptibility effect could increase the chances for chronic bronchitis and lung cancer.

Family History, Genetics, and Lung Cancer

Even if they are nonsmokers, people who have first-degree relatives (parents, children, or siblings) with lung cancer can have a higher risk for this illness. Although lung cancer is usually associated with smoking or other external factors, researchers have found clues suggesting that some people are more vulnerable to the disease.

A study of 52 families with a minimum of three first-degree family members with lung, throat, or laryngeal cancer found persuasive evidence for an inherited lung cancer susceptibility gene (or genes) on several chromosomes. What's more, the researchers found that while the noncarriers of the suspected familial lung cancer gene increased their risk for lung cancer the more they smoked, for the suspected carriers even a small amount of smoking increased their cancer risk. The results suggest that people with this potential familial lung cancer gene should be especially careful to avoid tobacco smoke.[24]

Radon Exposure

Colorless, odorless, and radioactive, radon gas is a toxic substance in the air and in some houses but most often underground. This means that miners and others who work within the earth are at a higher risk for radon exposure. Radon gas can inflict lung cell DNA damage directly, by inducing structural changes in genetic material or by bumping up the production of harmful reactive oxygen species that hurt DNA within cells.

Toxins in the Construction and Chemical Industries

Several compounds encountered in the construction and chemical industries also pose a lung cancer risk. These include asbestos, arsenic, nickel, soot, chromium, and tar. The longer a person has been exposed to these compounds, the higher that person's risk for lung cancer. The risk is greater yet for those who also smoke.

TOBACCO SMOKE AND LUNG CANCER

Tobacco smoke is, without a doubt, the most important risk factor for lung cancer as well as other cancers throughout the body. Thus the rest of this chapter examines the molecular mechanisms underlying tobacco smoke and cancer.

Lung cancer has been associated with smoking at least as far back as 1939, when a German doctor found that only 3 out of 86 patients with lung cancer were nonsmokers.[17] Since then, scientists have found many links between tobacco smoke and lung cancer. Researchers in 1950 conducted a broad epidemiological study on lung cancer patients and their smoking habits and determined that tobacco smoke had a positive association with lung cancer. They pointed to a strong relationship between lung cancer risk and amount of tobacco smoked.[1]

But it wasn't until 1964 that the U.S. surgeon general declared that smoking causes cancer. That report has had a huge impact on the public awareness of

tobacco-related issues such as addiction, use, and disease. It is now known that tobacco smoke causes a long list of diseases besides lung cancer, including cancers
of the bladder, cervix, esophagus, kidney, larynx, leukemia, mouth, and pancreas,
according to the National Cancer Institute.[25]

Studies have shown that women who smoke have a higher risk for infertility;
men who smoke have a higher risk for impotency. Pregnant smokers have double
the risk of a variety of complications for themselves and their babies, including
premature birth, low-birth-weight infants, and still births.[18]

While antismoking campaigns have reduced lung cancer incidence and mortality, young people are still lighting up. In the United States, estimates suggest
32 percent of grade 12 students smoke, while about 4,000 youths per day experiment with cigarettes (about half become habitual smokers).[19]

If current global smoking patterns continue, 1 billion deaths will be attributable
to tobacco use during the 21st century, with the death toll reaching 10 million per
year by 2030.[2]

Risk from Secondhand Tobacco Smoke

Also called environmental tobacco smoke or involuntary smoke, secondhand
smoke refers to the smoke rising off a burning cigarette as well as smokers' ex-
halations after puffing. This kind of tobacco smoke exposure is associated with
an increased risk for lung cancer as well as other diseases. In the United States,
secondhand smoke is blamed for about 3,000 lung cancer deaths and 35,000 coronary heart disease deaths among adult nonsmokers.[3]

Infants exposed to secondhand smoke are more at risk for sudden infant death
syndrome (SIDS), bronchitis, or pneumonia. People who work in occupations or
industries where smoking is permitted (or was permitted until recently) may have
high levels of secondhand smoke exposure and therefore an increased risk for
lung cancer and other illnesses. Some bars, restaurants, bowling alleys, pool halls,
casinos, and bingo parlors in the United States and other places still allow smoking. As secondhand smoke causes preventable death, more legislation is needed
to protect the public from this toxic exposure. Several U.S. states, European countries, and provinces in Canada have already banned smoking in restaurants and
other indoor public areas and workplaces.

Nicotine and Smoking

At the heart of the smoking problem is an addictive recreational drug: nicotine. An oily essence of tobacco, nicotine has been consumed in the Americas for
thousands of years. The ancients were diverse with their intake methods: tobacco
was chewed, sipped in tea, smoked, eaten, and inserted into the body via enemas.
All these techniques led to the absorption of nicotine, eventually identified by

scientists in the early 1800s. One of the most widely and heavily used drugs in the world today, nicotine has been shown by research to influence mood and behavior and is a powerfully addictive component of tobacco smoke.[5]

Cigarettes, as it turns out, are a very efficient delivery system for this drug—far more effective than chewing gum or applying skin patches, however much safer they may be to use. This is because inhaled tobacco smoke is quickly absorbed through lung tissue and reaches the brain in 7 to 10 seconds. It then produces a dramatic spike in blood serum nicotine levels—an effect that smokers crave. The results, however, last less than an hour. The number of cigarettes smoked per day is significant in terms of how much each smoker is exposed to nicotine and harmful compounds such as tar.[6] Many smokers commonly consume one to one and a half packs of cigarettes a day, puffing about 10 times on each cigarette. This means they will take in about one milligram of nicotine per cigarette, every day.

Scientists do not believe that nicotine causes the smoking-related cancers or respiratory diseases produced by other compounds in tobacco smoke, although some evidence suggests nicotine use leads to cardiovascular disease.

Nicotine Effects on the Brain and Addiction

Scientific studies have shown that when a person inhales cigarette smoke, the nicotine in the smoke is rapidly absorbed into the blood and produces many effects on the brain within seconds. Nicotine produces brain effects that are similar (although milder) to other habit-forming substances, including opiates, cocaine, and alcohol.

On the positive side, smokers may experience a better mood and a higher level of alertness, as well as learning and memory improvement, thanks to nicotine's stimulation of the dopaminergic pathways (the neural tracks in the brain where the neurotransmitter dopamine is sent from one area to another). Nicotine's actions on the brain also include mimicking a neurotransmitter molecule called acetylcholine, leading to the release of adrenaline, also known as the fight-or-flight hormone.[7] As a consequence, smokers experience a higher heart rate and blood pressure, less fatigue, less stress, a better mood, less hunger, and the easing of any withdrawal symptoms. As nicotine limits insulin secretion, less glucose is absorbed from the blood; at the same time, synthesis of the energy-balancing hormone neuropeptide Y in the brain may be impeded.[8] As a result, smokers usually have a little extra sugar in the blood (hyperglycemia), suppressing their hunger. Nicotine is a euphoriant, and it controls smokers' behavior by ensuring smokers avoid withdrawal.[9]

On the downside, nicotine's pleasing effects ease off quickly, within minutes in fact, so smokers must continue to dose themselves to maintain their feelings of well-being. Meanwhile, long-term nicotine exposure is suspected of increasing levels of unhealthy cholesterol in the blood, possibly leading to a higher risk of heart disease. Unfortunately, although people who quit smoking are taking great steps toward better health, stopping the regular supply of nicotine to their brains provokes a long list of unpleasant side effects, at least for the short term. These include irritability, distractibility, anger, restlessness, anxiety, a lowered heart rate, and hunger. Over time, they may also gain weight—most ex-smokers are heavier than the norm.

Tobacco, a Dirty Delivery System

Although the forms of tobacco in use today do not have breadth of the variety of those of our ancestors, people craving nicotine can choose pipes, cigars, chewing tobacco, dipping tobacco, flavored cigarettes, and hookahs. Cigarettes, however, are the most popular nicotine delivery system at present. They are considered a dirty delivery system as they have added flavorings or other chemicals to enhance nicotine's effects on the brain. This is in addition to the 3,000 compounds already present in tobacco—or the 4,000 compounds in tobacco smoke. A number of these substances are known carcinogens, some found to initiate or promote cancer, others discovered to combine with other carcinogens in toxic ways or attack the cells of specific organs.[10]

While nicotine addiction underlies smokers' compulsion to smoke, other compounds in tobacco smoke are responsible for most of the habit's bodily harm. Scientific investigation of tobacco industry documents has revealed that at least 100 of the nearly 600 documented tobacco additives act to mask the smell of environmental tobacco smoke, boost or maintain nicotine delivery, possibly enhance the addictiveness of cigarette tobacco, and hide symptoms and sicknesses linked to the smoking habit.[11]

Some of these added compounds are harmless flavorings such as dill seeds or vanilla, but others are not so benign. Smokers may also be inhaling ammonia and ammonia salts, ingredients found in home cleaning products and fertilizers. These compounds are thought to promote the addictiveness of nicotine. In fact, studies have shown that ammonia raises the pH value of tobacco, allowing more nicotine to be freed from the cells of tobacco leaves. Once heated, this nicotine becomes vapor and is more rapidly absorbed into the brain.[12]

The tobacco additive levulinic acid has several actions that manipulate the smoking experience: it boosts nicotine yields while making the smoke seem smoother and milder; lowers the pH of tobacco smoke (which makes the smoke less irritating to smokers' upper respiratory tracts so they can inhale more deeply); and pumps up nicotine's effect on the brain by binding the addictive substance to neurons that normally would not respond to nicotine.[13]

The tobacco additive glycyrrhizin, a food sweetener derived from licorice and cocoa, camouflages tobacco's bitterness but also functions as a bronchodilator that lets smokers inhale more smoke into their lungs. As an alkaloid, it has pharmacological qualities that may be useful medicinally but can be toxic otherwise.

Some of these additives become carcinogens when burned with tobacco. More needs to be known about other potentially harmful by-products of tobacco combustion.

Carcinogenic Compounds in Tobacco and Their Effects

Aside from the potential hazards of tobacco additives, a minimum of 63 of the 4,000 identified compounds in tobacco smoke are carcinogenic. Eleven of these cause cancer in people. The most toxic of this group include polycyclic aromatic hydrocarbons (PAHs) and tobacco-specific nitrosamines (TSNs). These carcinogens directly harm DNA in lung cells, leading to DNA mutations and an increased possibility of lung cancer. Thanks to experiments exposing normal cultured bronchial (lung) cells to PAHs, scientists have learned that the carcinogen's metabolites can produce DNA damage (adducts). Mutations matching this type of bronchial DNA damage have been found in lung cancer as well as in the nearby, noninvolved lung tissues in people who smoke.

Some studies show that these PAHs and TSNs harm DNA by inducing mutations in the $p53$ tumor suppressor gene.[15] This key gene helps prevent tumor growth by stopping cells with unrepaired DNA from dividing. When mutated, $p53$ may allow cells with damaged DNA to replicate, possibly leading to tumor growth and cancer. About 60 percent of all cases of lung cancer show this mutation—although it is found less often in the lung cancers of nonsmokers. This suggests that the $p53$ mutations may be caused by immediate damage to lung tissues by tobacco smoke carcinogens rather than by preexisting mutations within the lung tissue.

How much harm carcinogens will do to any particular individual depends on a number of factors: the number of tobacco exposures daily, the type of tobacco smoke inhaled, the smoker's metabolism, and the health and effectiveness of his or her DNA repair mechanisms. It also matters how early a smoker began the habit, the degree of smoke inhalation, and the quality and quantity of various tobacco factors such as amounts of tar and nicotine and type of filter.[14]

Harmful Gases and Tar Particles in Tobacco Smoke

Those white streams of tobacco smoke rising off burning cigarettes or emerging from smokers' lungs are, in fact, clouds of gases and condensed tar particles. According to some estimates, 150 billion tar particles per cubic inch of tobacco are released through tobacco smoke. Gases toxic to bodily tissues included in this harmful fog are nitrogen oxide and carbon monoxide. As a person smokes, various undesirable effects begin. The tar and toxic gases fill the respiratory tract, irritating tissues, overstimulating mucous secretion, and injuring the smallest structures of lung tissue, the alveoli. The smoker's blood and tissues are deprived of oxygen as carbon monoxide attaches to hemoglobin, preventing oxygen delivery. If the smoker continues to maintain high levels of carbon monoxide in the blood, arteries become hardened, ultimately causing a predisposition to heart disease.

Other poisonous gases inhaled during a puff include formaldehyde, acrolein, hydrogen cyanide, and nitrogen oxides. Some of these are known human carcinogens. Meanwhile, the tar particles, representing 5 to 8 percent of the total emissions from a cigarette, clog up lung tissues and thus lower lung efficiency. The smoker becomes more vulnerable to chronic infection, chronic bronchitis, emphysema, and eventually, lung cancer.

CIGAR SMOKING

Cigar smoking has become more popular recently, probably in part due to images in the media of glamorous celebrities blithely puffing on stogies. Glossy magazines such as *Cigar Aficionado* have helped polish the image of cigar smokers as wealthy and worldly sophisticates—an image often held by smokers and nonsmokers alike. For many, cigars represent the good life.

But are cigars as harmful as cigarettes? The answer is yes—and no. A few key differences exist between cigars and cigarettes. The U.S. Department of Treasury defines cigars as any cake of tobacco wrapped in leaf tobacco or in any tobacco-containing substance. Cigarettes are defined as any roll of tobacco enclosed in paper or any tobaccoless material. But the main difference between the two nicotine delivery systems is how the tobacco is processed.

Cigars are assembled without filters and are made from air-cured and fermented tobaccos. U.S. cigarettes have filters and are made with a mix of mostly heat-cured and air-cured tobaccos with some sun-cured tobacco added in, but they contain no fermented tobacco. This is significant because the method of processing cigar tobacco makes the dried mix high in worrisome carcinogens. Fermenting tobacco may improve its smell and taste, but the process reduces nitrite to nitrate, which can react with various tobacco constituents to form more potent N-nitrosating nitrites. This compound responds to amines by forming carcinogens called nitrosamines.

Compared to cigarettes, cigars are also richer in the carcinogenic N-nitrosonornicotine, tobacco-specific carcinogens. Because of fermentation, levels of cigar tobacco protein, sugars, phytosterols, and polyphenols are lower than those in cigarette tobacco. Thus, cigar smoke contains generous amounts of nitrogen oxides, nitrosamines, and ammonia. Cigar smoke's higher pH means it also more readily dissolves in saliva, thereby freeing up more nicotine.

Research shows cigar smoke contains more tobacco-specific nitrosamines than cigarette smoke. However, a study compared amounts of tar, nicotine, and carbon monoxide in various manufactured and hand-rolled Canadian cigarettes and in small and large cigars. The scientists found the highest levels of tar, nicotine, and carbon monoxide in the smoke of small cigars. The next worst were hand-rolled and regular cigarettes. The big cigars had the lowest amounts of these toxins.[16]

The results indicate that the amount of tar and toxic gases in cigar smoke depends on the type of cigar smoked and that some cigarettes may pose a greater risk for lung diseases and cancer than some cigars.

Cigar versus Cigarette Smoke

Very little research has focused on cigar smoke; instead much of the scientific knowledge of tobacco and its smoke has been gathered from studies on cigarettes. The chemistry of both types of tobacco smoke is thought to be similar, aside from characteristics created by the chemicals added to cigarettes (mostly) or by cigar tobacco fermentation.

Dissimilarities in quality are likely caused by the different smoke pH and oxygen concentration levels. These, in turn, are due to the qualities of the tobacco wrapper versus the porous cigarette paper wrapper. Ultimately, tossing the cigarettes in favor of smoking large cigars may not reduce one's chances of tobacco-related cancer. Cigarette and cigar smokers have similar chances of developing cancers of the mouth and esophagus, areas of first contact with tobacco smoke.[20]

Tobacco Smoke as Environmental Pollutant

Rising from a cigar, cigarette, or pipe or exhaled by a smoker, the gases produced from burning tobacco add significant pollutants to the environment. These unwelcome substances include carbon monoxide; nitrogen oxides; various small, potentially harmful particles that can be inhaled (respirable suspended particulate matter); nicotine; and PAHs. A study measuring pollutants from tobacco smoke at cigar parties and at the homes of cigar smokers found levels of carbon monoxide that matched levels found on busy freeways in California.[20]

At peak levels, one cigar party had particulate pollution at levels that equaled a bustling parking garage, or 10 parts per million over a nearly three-and-a-half-hour event. Meanwhile, the outside rush-hour carbon monoxide level was a much lower 2 parts per million or less. The Environmental Protection Agency puts the maximum permissible level of carbon monoxide at 9 parts per million over eight hours.

Genetic Factors to Addiction

It's an old question: why do some people become addicted to various substances and others not? It appears that nicotine addiction is connected to how quickly the drug is metabolized, as the rate determines its effect on smokers.

Furthermore, evidence has been found for a genetic factor in nicotine addiction, thanks to studies of genetic variations in the part of the brain that regulates pleasure and reward, the dopaminergic signaling pathway.

People with mutations in the genes that encode for enzymes that assist with nicotine metabolism and neurotransmitter synthesis, the cytochrome *p450* gene family, are considered to have a genetic influence regarding the smoking habit. Some people with particular gene variations can metabolize nicotine faster and with fewer ill effects (such as headache and nausea) than people without the gene variation and thus may be more likely to become habitual smokers. On the other hand, others have what is considered an inactive variant of the gene and metabolize nicotine much more slowly. They are less likely to become addicted to tobacco smoke as the unpleasant side effects may put them off the habit.

According to other studies, some people may have genetic mutations in the dopamine pathway that affect their vulnerability to nicotine dependence. Those who have fewer binding sites in the brain for dopamine (dopamine receptors) have a greater chance of becoming addicted to tobacco smoke. Scientists theorize that some smokers may be using nicotine to compensate for their lack of dopamine receptors.

In the future, this information may be used to design antismoking treatments in a way that best suits smokers' genes.[21]

SUMMARY

Tobacco smoke is the number-one human carcinogen—and the leading cause of preventable death. This carcinogen has been well established as a factor in a long list of diseases and cancers, including lung, oral, esophageal, and bladder cancer. A variety of health risks exist whether the tobacco is in cigarette, cigar, or smokeless chewable, or inhalable (snuff) forms.

In cigarettes, not only do the tar and toxic gases produced by burning tobacco injure the lung tissues but many of the nearly 600 tobacco additives can also do serious harm. Among these additives are compounds you would ordinarily bring nowhere near your mouth, including ammonia. Some of these compounds or their by-products are known carcinogens that induce tumor growth in laboratory animals. More research and regulation is needed to limit harm that may be caused by these compounds.

Other causes for lung cancer are not quite as clear-cut and may not be as preventable, considering new Human Genome Project research that suggests some people may carry a gene that increases their risk for the disease. In fact several mutations have been identified as associated with an increased risk for lung cancer, and several genes are now implicated in gene susceptibility.[22] Anyone who suspects a familial susceptibility toward lung cancer should of course take great care to avoid all forms of tobacco smoke and other lung irritants and damaging substances such as radon, air pollution, asbestos, and cooking fumes. Genetic counseling may also be a consideration.

Chapter 12

Ovarian and Endometrial Cancers

Ovarian cancer strikes fewer than half as many women as endometrial cancer, yet ovarian cancer has double the mortality rate. Comparing these two female-specific cancers illustrates a powerful point: early detection is the key to successful outcomes.

OVARIAN CANCER

Ovarian cancer is the fifth-most-common gynecological cancer and is found almost exclusively in postmenopausal women. As its name suggests, ovarian cancer forms in ovary tissues, usually either in the egg cells or in cells lining the ovary's surface. According to the National Cancer Institute, an estimated 21,880 women in the United States were diagnosed with ovarian cancer in 2010. About 13,850 died from the disease that same year.[16]

Although ovarian cancer is one of the less common cancers, it is the most deadly of the female-specific cancers. This is because most women don't receive a diagnosis until the cancer has reached an advanced stage. Sadly, no effective screening tests can offer an early detection for ovarian cancer.

Ovarian Cancer Symptoms

The symptoms for this cancer tend to be vague at first. As the disease progresses, women may experience discomfort or pressure in their pelvic area, back, abdomen or legs. They may feel fatigued, bloated, nauseated, constipated, and have diarrhea or indigestion. Some women experience breathlessness, vaginal bleeding—even after menopause—and feel they have to urinate frequently.

ENDOMETRIAL CANCER

Endometrial cancer (also known as uterine cancer) develops in the tissue lining the uterus. This disease is a few steps ahead of ovarian cancer in terms of how frequently it is diagnosed, but it tends to be much less deadly. The numbers tell part of the story: in 2010, about 43,470 women in the United States were diagnosed with endometrial cancer and an estimated 7,950 died from it.[10] Fewer women die from endometrial cancer than ovarian cancer as early symptoms for endometrial cancer are much more obvious.

Endometrial Cancer Symptoms

Women with early-stage endometrial cancer may experience unexplained vaginal spotting or bleeding between menstrual periods or after menopause (when they should not experience any bleeding). They may have pain or difficulty during urination, discomfort during sex, or pain in the pelvic region.

The rest of this chapter will examine these two female-specific cancers separately, beginning with ovarian cancer.

OVARIAN CANCER RISK FACTORS

Age is a risk factor: most women diagnosed with ovarian cancer are older than age 55. Very few women with ovarian cancer are younger than age 40. Women who started menstruating at an early age are thought to have a slightly higher risk for ovarian cancer. Those who suffered from infertility or who never had children are also believed to have an increased risk. Some evidence shows that the more ovulation cycles a woman experiences in her life, the greater her chance for ovarian cancer.[8,9] However, women who have multiple pregnancies, breastfeed their children, experience early menopause, and used birth control pills have a reduced risk for ovarian cancer. This suggests that reproductive factors have a relationship to ovarian cancer risk.

Some research indicates that hormones play a role in ovarian cancer development, as women who take estrogen without progesterone in hormone therapy for menopause for more than a decade have a higher ovarian cancer risk. Studies have also shown a mildly increased ovarian cancer risk with obesity, the use of talcum powder, and specific fertility drugs, although some of the information is inconsistent. Other ovarian cancer risk factors include exposure to ionizing radiation, chemical carcinogens, family history, and personal cancer history (especially for women who have had cancer of the rectum, colon, uterus, or breast). Lifestyle choices such as smoking and certain dietary patterns are also suspected to contribute to increase risk of ovarian cancer.

Diet and Ovarian Cancer Risk

Diet is a potential key factor in ovarian cancer risk. Observational research featuring long-term nutritional assessments in different countries focused on links between dietary patterns and ovarian cancer. In general, the data point to a strong connection between total fat (all fat sources) or animal fat consumption and ovarian cancer risk. The conclusion is that switching to vegetable fat from animal fat may reduce ovarian cancer risk.[1]

High fat consumption, particularly animal fats, may stimulate the body to make more estrogen hormone, which in turn may increase ovulation, thereby increasing ovarian cancer risk. For example, women who regularly eat large servings of eggs have a higher risk for ovarian cancer. Women who habitually dine on high-fiber foods and green leafy vegetables, however, have a lower risk for ovarian cancer.[2] Other dietary studies have concluded that women who eat generous amounts of vegetables reduce their risk for this cancer. Diets high in fruit do not appear to have any particular benefits regarding ovarian cancer risk.[3]

Hormones, Growth Factors, and Ovarian Cancer

A noted earlier, a higher risk for ovarian cancer appears to be linked to the frequency of ovulation, as well as women's infertility or nulliparity (never given birth), while a reduced risk is associated with giving birth to several children as well as breastfeeding. By these facts alone it seems that limiting one's exposure to female sex hormones (such as ovulation-stimulating estrogens and estradiol metabolites; that are intermediates and products of estradiol metabolism) may have a protective effect against ovarian cancer.

More evidence for the link between long-term female sex hormone exposure and ovarian cancer comes from cell culture studies. Researchers found that some estradiol metabolites have a strong stimulating effect on ovarian cancer cells.[4]

The ovaries produce two main hormones, estrogen and progesterone, that shift in dominance during the female monthly cycle. These hormonal changes help ensure the proper functioning of the female reproductive system. Scientists believe that when the balance of the sex hormones shifts toward more estrogen, the risk for ovarian cancer rises. This may be why postmenopausal hormone replacement therapy may make some women more susceptible to ovarian cancer.[4]

Researchers do not know exactly what function progesterone plays in regard to the development of ovarian cancer but suspect this hormone helps prevent cancer. This is also suggested by studies that show a link between ovarian cancer and women who take estrogen alone, versus the combination of estrogen and progestin therapy.

Growth Factors and Ovarian Cancer

Growth factors are proteins that regulate cell growth and metabolism. They play a critical role in the development of ovarian cancer. Some research has demonstrated that levels of the insulin-like growth factor binding protein-2 (IGFBP-2) are higher in women with advanced epithelial ovarian cancers compared to controls and women with noncancerous gynecological diseases. Serum levels of the growth factor are also higher in women with early to advanced ovarian cancer. This study's results support the theory that the insulin-like growth factor pathway may be a key player in the development of epithelial ovarian cancer, possibly by enhancing the proliferation of ovarian cells.[5] IGFBP-2 is an important biomarker that can indicate metabolic disorders such as obesity and may well be an indicator for sedentary- or obesity-related association with a higher risk for ovarian cancer. Other research has not found a positive link between insulin-like growth-factor-related proteins and ovarian cancer risk, however.[6]

Genetic Predisposition

Germ-line mutations in genes thought to increase the risk for cancers of the breast, prostate, and pancreas are also linked to a familial predisposition to ovarian cancer. These key mutations are found on the *BRCA*1 and *BRCA*2 genes and are very rare. In most communities, fewer than 1 in 500 people carries this gene, except in the Ashkenazi Jewish population. In this group, 1 out of 40 people carries the mutation. Although less than 10 percent of women with ovarian cancer have the inherited genetic predisposition, for high-risk families these identified mutations have important implications regarding genetic counseling and testing. The *BRCA*1 and *BRCA*2 genes encode proteins that, among other duties, are thought to assist in DNA repair. This is important as studies show that flaws in the repair mechanisms for damaged DNA underlie cancer development and progression.[11,12]

Lynch Syndrome

A familial condition, Lynch syndrome is also known as hereditary nonpolyposis colorectal cancer (HNPCC) and is caused by an abnormality in a gene responsible for DNA repair. Women with this disease have a 10 to 12 percent risk of ovarian cancer in their lifetime, as well as an increased risk for endometrial cancer and colorectal cancer. Women with Lynch syndrome develop a type of ovarian cancer that is clinically different from the ovarian cancer found in women without the inherited condition. Most importantly, ovarian cancer develops at a much younger age in these women—about a third develop ovarian cancer before age 40 and half are diagnosed between the ages of 40 and 50.[7]

Scientific studies suggest that removing the uterus (prophylactic hysterectomy) with the ovaries and fallopian tubes (bilateral salpingo-oophorectomy) is an effective strategy for preventing endometrial and ovarian cancer in women with Lynch syndrome.[7]

Ionizing Radiation

Ionizing radiation is linked to a higher risk of ovarian cancer. High rates of ovarian cancer were noted in Japanese women who had been exposed to radiation from the atomic bomb blast in World War II, as well as in women who received pelvic irradiation for cervical cancer and noncancerous diseases.[13,14]

Ovarian Cancer and Endometriosis

A genetic disorder that increases the risk for ovarian cancer, endometriosis is a common disease caused when cells normally found within the uterus migrate to other areas in the body. Women with this condition often experience infertility and pelvic pain. Although the risk factors associated with endometriosis are not well established, suspected risk factors include genetic abnormalities and environmental, immunological, angiogenic, and endocrine processes. Although endometriosis is a benign disorder, recent studies of endometriosis suggest that this condition is associated with endometrial cancer and ovarian cancer.[15]

ENDOMETRIAL CANCER RISK FACTORS

As with ovarian cancer, excessive exposure to estrogen is also a risk factor for endometrial cancer. The hormone and its metabolites can stimulate the endometrium to grow, possibly predisposing the organ tissue to endometrial cancer. As early-onset menstruation increases levels of estrogen in the body, women who began their menstrual cycles before age 12 and who continued to menstruate into their 50th years have a higher risk for endometrial cancer. Scientists believe that the more years of menstruation a woman has, the more frequently her endometrium is exposed to estrogen's growth-provoking effects.

Women who have not had children also have a higher risk of endometrial cancer. During pregnancy, progesterone levels rise in the mother's body while estrogen levels decrease—offering the mother a protective effect against endometrial cancer.

Another risk factor for this cancer is irregular ovulation, also known as polycystic ovary syndrome (PCOS).

Obesity, Diabetes, and Endometrial Cancer

Ovaries are one source of estrogen; body fat is another. As fat tissues can induce estrogen production (and that of other hormones), having excess body fat can mean higher levels of estrogen in the body. This in turn can lead to a raised risk for endometrial and ovarian cancers, among others. Eating high-fat foods may promote obesity and thus spark more estrogen production, but some researchers also believe these rich, greasy foods may have a direct impact on estrogen metabolism, thereby increasing the risk for endometrial cancer. As diabetes often accompanies obesity, it is also considered a risk for endometrial cancer—although some research has demonstrated that even overweight women with diabetes have a raised risk for endometrial cancer.

Again, as with ovarian cancer, estrogen-only replacement therapy for post-menopausal women may stimulate endometrium growth and increase the chances for endometrial cancer. But if these same women take synthetic progestin combined with estrogen in their hormone replacement therapy, they may lower their risk for endometrial cancer—although other health risks may increase. Ovarian tumors themselves may also be sources of estrogen that bump up the body's estrogen levels. It is not unusual for endometrial cancers to develop from benign endometrial abnormalities. The good news is that doctors often can find these abnormalities during routine examinations and offer treatment before they become cancerous.

SUMMARY

Comparing incidence and mortality rates between these two gynecological diseases illustrates the importance of early diagnosis and treatment of ovarian and endometrial cancers. Therefore, all women should ensure they have regular gynecological examinations, especially if they are among those in the higher risk groups.

Some women may consider genetic counseling and testing if they believe they are carrying a high-risk gene mutation or have one of the familial diseases that predispose them to cancer.

Chapter 13

Pancreatic Cancer

As its mortality rate nearly equals its incidence rate, pancreatic cancer is one of the deadliest cancers known. Also called exocrine pancreatic cancer (the most common form of pancreatic cancer), this disease killed an estimated 281,000 people around the world in 2010, according to the International Agency for Research on Cancer.[15] In the United States alone, in 2010 about 43,140 new cases of pancreatic cancer were diagnosed, according to the National Cancer Institute.[16] That same year, about 36,800 people across the country died from the illness. All in all, fewer than 4 percent of people with pancreatic cancer survive past five years with the illness. In fact, most people with pancreatic cancer die within one to two years of diagnosis.[1]

Part of the reason for this disease's heavy mortality rate is due to the pancreas's hard-to-reach location, tucked in behind the stomach and next to the small intestine. This cone-shaped gland secretes digestive juices and insulin as well as other hormones, but it is difficult to access using conventional endoscopic screening tools. Early detection and therapeutic intervention for pancreatic cancer lags behind the treatment for other cancer diseases for several other reasons as well: Pancreatic cancer tends to be diagnosed in its later stages as the illness has few obvious early indicators. Because of its proximity to other major organs, such as the bile ducts and vital vascular structures, surgery on the organ becomes complicated. Pancreatic cancer cells tend to resist chemotherapy and radiotherapy treatments. This cancer is therefore known as one of the greatest challenges in oncology.

More common to the Western world than in developing countries, pancreatic cancer's highest incidence rates are in the United States. That said, this disease is still one of the rarer forms of cancer, accounting for less than 2 percent of cancer-related deaths in the United States, but because of its aggressiveness, pancreatic cancer is the fourth-most-common cause of death from cancer.

SYMPTOMS

As noted above, part of the reason why pancreatic cancer is so deadly is that this disease has no clear early symptoms. But as the disease progresses, people with pancreatic cancer may experience pain in the upper abdomen or upper back, weakness, a decreased appetite, nausea and vomiting, weight loss, and the yellowed skin, eyes, and darkened urine of jaundice. While these symptoms are not sure signs of pancreatic cancer and could instead indicate another health problem, anyone with these symptoms should consult with a doctor as soon as possible.

RISK FACTORS

The very few established risk factors for pancreatic cancer also tend to be associated with other cancer diseases. These include tobacco smoke, age, gender (men have higher incidence rates than women), ethnicity (African Americans have the highest incidence rates), genetic susceptibility, personal and family cancer history, chronic pancreatitis, diabetes, obesity, and various occupational exposures. More detail on these factors follows in this chapter. Other possible risk factors such as physical inactivity and gall bladder disease are not firmly established due to a lack of research or inconsistent data.[2]

Age, Gender, and Ethnicity

The data show that the risk for pancreatic cancer is very rare in people younger than age 30 but increases sharply with passing years. Peak years of incidence are between ages 70 and 80. Overall, more men get pancreatic cancer and die from it than women, and this is true around the world. In the United States, African Americans are more prone to this disease than Asian Americans, Hispanics, or Caucasians.

Tobacco Smoke

Tobacco smoke appears to be the most significant risk factor with respect to pancreatic cancer. Men and women who smoke tobacco, particularly heavy smokers, have double the risk of nonsmokers developing pancreatic cancer, according to some studies.[11,12] Smokers have a higher risk for lung cancer (about 15 times that of nonsmokers' risk) than pancreatic cancer as their lungs are directly exposed to smoke; the pancreas, meanwhile, receives tobacco smoke carcinogens less directly.

In smokers the pancreas comes in contact with tobacco-related carcinogens via the bloodstream or through pancreatic exposure to bile or duodenal contents. Most pancreatic cancers develop in the area known as the head of the gland, an area that could be exposed to tobacco carcinogens in duodenal fluid or bile.[3]

Genetic Predisposition, Family History, and Chronic Pancreatitis

Some people are genetically predisposed to having chronic inflammation in their pancreas, a condition called chronic pancreatitis that can greatly increase the risk for pancreatic cancer. Chronic pancreatitis develops when digestive enzymes secreted by the pancreas (and intended for the small intestine) mistakenly become active inside the pancreas. As a result, the enzymes begin digesting the pancreas. Repeated acute attacks of this painful condition cause scarring. Tobacco smoke exposure is a risk factor for chronic pancreatitis, as are excessive alcohol consumption and *H. pylori* infection.[5] Scientists suspect that the persistent and chronic inflammation of pancreatitis somehow induces or promotes the development of pancreatic cancer. But pancreatitis is a rare disease and can be linked to only about 4 percent of pancreatic cancer patients.

However, chronic pancreatitis can cause problems regarding food digestion, due to a lack of digestive enzymes. This condition, called endocrine pancreatic dysfunction, can lead to a secondary form of diabetes. While this type of diabetes amounts for less than 1 percent of all diabetes cases, 80 percent of people with chronic pancreatitis will develop diabetes—itself an important risk factor for death in patients with chronic pancreatitis.[6]

Familial Pancreatic Cancer

Familial predisposition to pancreatic cancer amounts to less than 10 percent of total cases, but if you have a parent or sibling with pancreatic cancer, your risk for this disease triples. In fact, some studies have reported the increased risk as up to five times that of the general population for first-degree relatives of people with pancreatic cancer.

Yet while this risk factor has been well established, scientists have not found a gene responsible for this familial component to pancreatic cancer risk. The closest are the mutations in the inherited *BRCA1* and *BRCA2* genes linked to other cancers such as familial breast, ovarian, and prostate cancers. These mutated genes may also contribute to pancreatic cancer. *BRCA1* and *BRCA2* are tumor suppressor genes that help prevent cells with damaged DNA from replicating before they are repaired. If mutated, they may not function correctly to prevent damaged cells from dividing. As these mutations are seen in other types of familial cancers, some researchers believe these genes are important regulatory genes. These mutations have also been linked to sporadic pancreatic cancer.

Other inherited diseases that are linked to an increased risk for pancreatic cancer include hereditary pancreatitis (see above), hereditary nonpolyposis colorectal cancer (HNPCC), Peutz-Jeghers syndrome, and familial atypical multiple mole melanoma (FAMMM) syndrome. These familial syndromes that are accompanied by an increased risk for pancreatic cancer are rare, accounting for a small percentage of familial pancreatic cancer cases. The search continues for the gene or genes responsible for the genetic component of pancreatic cancer.[1,4]

Occupational Exposure

So far, researchers have not been able to consistently point at any particular occupation as a high-risk environment for pancreatic cancer. Instead, some compounds are suspected to be involved in the progression of this disease. These include chlorinated hydrocarbons (CHCs), found in the rubber and plastic manufacturing industries, chemical plants, the pharmaceutical industry, dry cleaning, paint removal, the metal industry, and various laboratories. Several known or suspected human carcinogens include the CHC-related polychlorinated biphenyls (PCBs), vinyl chloride, and CHC solvents.

Additionally, some pesticides may be involved in the development of pancreatic cancer, including DDT (dichlorodiphenyltrichloroethane), but it seems unlikely these play a role in causing the cancer.[8]

Obesity, Diabetes, and Pancreatic Cancer

In recent years, studies have linked obesity and type 2 diabetes with a higher risk for pancreatic cancer, although some of the data conflict regarding diabetes's connection. (Type 1 diabetes, also known as juvenile diabetes, is not associated with an increased risk for pancreatic cancer.) Several studies have investigated whether diabetes is a risk factor for the development or progression of pancreatic cancer but found no conclusive evidence. Whether diabetes could cause or is a consequence of pancreatic cancer development needs to be established in a large-population study.[13,14]

Some scientific reports show that a link between type 2 diabetes and pancreatic cancer could be due to a diet high in sugar and high-sugar foods. This could induce frequent hyperglycemia, increase insulin demand, and decrease insulin sensitivity.[7] As one of the pancreas's primary roles is to release the hormones glucagon and insulin in the blood so blood glucose can be used for energy, a high-sugar diet would keep the pancreas busy secreting hormones. Thus people who eat too much sugar and who may be overweight often develop metabolic problems that may contribute to developing diabetes. These include insulin resistance, abnormal glucose metabolism (hyperinsulinemia), and impaired glucose tolerance.

Unlike diabetes type 1 (usually seen in young people who have developed insulin insufficiency), diabetes type 2 typically develops in overweight adults who have adopted an inactive lifestyle. While diabetes type 2 has been reliably linked with a higher risk for pancreatic cancer, the relationship between the diseases is puzzling. This is because some people become diabetic as a manifestation of an underlying pancreatic tumor. Generally, when this is the case, the patient develops diabetes suddenly, and a few months later pancreatic cancer is found.

Diet

As the incidence of pancreatic cancer varies greatly around the globe, multiple studies have investigated how diet and lifestyle factors affect pancreatic cancer risk.

Tobacco smoking is a key risk factor for pancreatic cancer, and its popularity in some countries is one explanation for higher incidence of the disease. Some research has demonstrated that higher total calories and, possibly, higher levels of dietary fat could also lead to an increased risk for pancreatic cancer.

The food preservatives nitrites (NO_2) and nitrates (NO_3) are also associated with pancreatic cancer because when eaten, these compounds can become potent carcinogens called nitrosamines. Other studies show that when combined with gastric or duodenal acidity, the N-nitrosamines or N-nitrosamides (from food, tobacco smoke, or chemicals) can increase the chances for pancreatic cancer.[9,10] On the positive side, some researchers theorize that the antioxidants from fruit and vegetables may prevent toxic substances from harming the pancreas, thereby reducing the risk of pancreatic cancer.

SUMMARY

Pancreatic cancer is sometimes called a "silent disease" because it offers no clear warning symptoms in its early stages. It is also notoriously difficult to treat. Located in an awkward place inside the body, very close to major digestive organs, surgery in this area is problematical. The disease is also resistant to chemotherapy and radiation.

Because diabetes appears to increase the risk for pancreatic cancer, it is perhaps not surprising that weight gain and an inactive lifestyle are also associated with a higher risk. Exercise, however, and a diet featuring plenty of fruit and vegetables is thought to protect against pancreatic cancer.

Although research has shown smoking to be the most dangerous risk factor for pancreatic cancer, most studies indicate that the extra risk from smoking disappears within a decade of smoking cessation, regardless of the amount of cigarettes smoked daily or yearly.

Chapter 14

Prostate Cancer

This very common disease is the second-leading cause of cancer death in U.S. men, and all men face the risk of developing this cancer. About 32,000 men in the United States were expected to die from this disease in 2010, while about 218,000 were newly diagnosed that same year, according to figures from the National Cancer Institute.[16]

But in spite of the pervasiveness of this disease, its risk factors are not well understood. So far, only age, family history, and ethnicity are considered prostate cancer risk factors. Researchers suspect that other possible factors involved in the disease include exposure to sex steroid hormones, sexually transmitted diseases, inflammation, excess body weight, and low levels of vitamin D. Some studies have focused on other potential factors such as tobacco smoke, diabetes, and alcohol use, but no clear ties to or roles in the disease process were found.[1]

SYMPTOMS

A gland in the male reproductive system, the prostate is located internally, below the bladder and in front of the rectum. Thus early symptoms often have to do with the urinary tract. Men with prostate cancer will often have difficulty urinating or stopping the flow of urine. They may need to urinate often, frequently at night, and experience a burning or otherwise painful feeling during the process. They may have trouble getting an erection, find blood in their urine or semen, and often have pain in the lower back region, hips, or upper thighs. It is important to note that these symptoms may also be caused by other health problems, such as prostatitis. However, men with these symptoms should see their urologist as soon as possible; when detected early, prostate cancer is curable.

RISK FACTORS

Age

Age is the least understood of all the possible causes of prostate cancer. While prostate cancer is rarely found in anyone younger than age 50, and the chances of getting prostate cancer rise with age (most American men with prostate cancer are 65 years old or older), these characteristics are changing. Younger men are increasingly diagnosed with this cancer.[2]

Racial and Ethnic Variation

Geographic origin or ethnicity has a clear connection to men's risk for prostate cancer, although scientists are not certain why. African American men have the highest incidence for prostate cancer in the world. They are one and half times as likely as Caucasian Americans and Hispanic Americans to get this cancer and three times as likely as men of Asian origin. African American men are also more likely to die of this disease than men of other ethnicities. Asian men who live in their countries of origin have the lowest risks in the world.

The change in risk for immigrants suggests environmental factors may be significant to this disease. For example, second and third generations of men of Chinese origin living in the United States who have adopted a Western diet have a significantly higher risk for prostate cancer than men in China.[3] In general, the incidence for prostate cancer is lowest in developing countries and highest in Western countries.

Several studies, however, report higher incidence and mortality rates for prostate cancer for African men in their native African countries than for African Americans. The most important finding to date on this issue is the discovery of genetic mutations that are associated with increased prostate cancer risk in men with African ancestry.[13,14,15]

Hereditary and Genetic Factors

While family links are not well understood, scientists believe some families have a familial, or hereditary, predisposition to prostate cancer. The research suggests men who have a father or brother with prostate cancer may have as much as twice the risk of developing the disease. The risk climbs higher when men have several close relatives with the disease, especially if their relatives were diagnosed at a young age. Men with distant relatives with prostate cancer have only a small increase in risk.

Scientists have found not one specific gene but several that increase prostate cancer risk. It may be that no single dominant genetic mutation is needed to develop this cancer. Researchers have noted that mutations in genes responsible for innate immune response are often seen in prostate cancer cells. These genetic changes may leave cells unable to defend themselves against infections, ultimately giving rise to chronic inflammation—one of the well-established risk factors for prostate cancer.

It is possible that the gene mutations only increase prostate cancer risk when another particular risk factor is present, such as a viral infection or an exposure to an environmental toxin. These factors may be different from population to population, offering one explanation for the differing prostate cancer risks.[4]

Mutations in two tumor suppressor genes, *Pten* and *p53*, are also thought to increase prostate cancer risk. Normally, these two genes encode for proteins that stop cells with damaged DNA from dividing, but when mutated, these genes may not be able to perform this key function. Thus, mutations in the *Pten* and *p53* genes remove the necessary cell proliferation control and may assist the initiation or progression of prostate cancer.

Another key gene that may be involved in prostate cancer is a carcinogen detoxifier called glutathione *S*-transferase. When normal, it protects cells from oxidative genome damage. When mutated, this gene becomes inactive—a form often found in prostate cancer. An inactive carcinogen detoxifier can leave cells vulnerable to carcinogens and other toxins or harmful compounds.

Prostate tumors are influenced by androgens (male sex hormones such as testosterone and dihydrotestosterone), therefore any alterations in genes involved in steroid hormone biosynthesis and metabolism may play a role in prostate disease. Some evidence shows ethnic variations regarding how frequently genes involved in androgen pathways are mutated. This may provide an explanation for the different incidence of prostate cancer among men of different ethnicities.[5]

Diet

Researchers observe that men who eat large amounts of fat, especially animal fat from red meat, put themselves at a significantly higher risk for prostate cancer. Fat incites the production of testosterone, which in turn boosts prostate cell growth. It should be no surprise, then, that prostate cancer is common in Western countries where dairy foods and meat are consumed regularly. On that note, a low incidence of prostate cancer is found in Asian countries, where the commonly eaten foods include rice, vegetables, and soybean products and very little red meat. As noted in the beginning of this chapter, Asian men are the least likely to develop prostate cancer, as long as they live in Asia. This further supports diet, particularly the Western diet, as a risk factor for prostate cancer.

High fat consumption appears to be the main dietary risk factor for many cancers, as well as prostate cancer. Most scientific research has focused on total, saturated, or animal fats, and although some findings are mixed, the results show a potential positive link between these fats and prostate cancer risk, as well as an inverse association with omega-3 fat. The findings are not so consistent regarding polyunsaturated fat, however.

Men who eat a lot of meat, red meat and processed meat in particular, are also at a higher risk for prostate cancer. Scientists, however, do not know if the increased risk is due to meat's high fat content, the carcinogens (such as nitrosamines) formed during high-temperature cooking methods, animal proteins, or as yet undiscovered factors.

The research also shows that men who eat plenty of fruit and vegetables rich in the antioxidant lycopene, such as tomatoes, pink grapefruit, and watermelon, may have a lower risk of prostate cancer. Other foods thought to be protective include the antioxidant-rich cruciferous vegetables (cabbage, broccoli, and cauliflower, for example) and allium vegetables (such as onions and garlic).[6]

Hormonal Influence

Male sex hormones, or androgens, are needed to develop male reproductive organs, such as the prostate. However, the research shows these hormones can also kick-start prostate cancer. Scientists note that male humans and male dogs castrated before reaching sexual maturation do not develop prostate cancer. But laboratory rats given testosterone will get the disease, as androgens encourage cell proliferation and prevent cell death.[10,11,12]

It is not clear whether ethnic variation in male sex hormone levels can explain the differences in prostate cancer risk between men of different geographic origin. Some researchers believe high levels of circulating testosterone and low levels of circulating estrogen metabolite (estradiol) may raise the risk for this disease.[6]

Otherwise, the steroid hormone vitamin D (manufactured in the body from sunlight exposure), may be significant in respect to ethnic variation. This vitamin may have antiproliferative, prodifferentiative, and proapoptotic effects on prostate cancer cells. Vitamin D also impedes tumor growth. However, some studies have shown ethnic variation in serum vitamin D levels. Low levels of serum vitamin D found in African American men may be connected to their higher risk for prostate cancer. As vitamin D production usually depends on sun exposure, people with more skin pigmentation and with possible genetic alterations relevant to the vitamin D production process may have lower circulating levels of vitamin D.[5] The result may be a higher risk for prostate cancer.

Chronic Inflammation

Inflammation is a tool the body uses to draw attention to cellular injury as well as stimulate the removal of irreparably harmed cells, infection, and foreign particles. When the immune system is unable to rid the body of bacteria, viruses, or some other irritating agent, inflammation can become chronic. Researchers believe chronic inflammation may be in part responsible for about one-quarter of all cancers. Various exposures may cause the initial irritation: dietary carcinogens, environmental toxins, or infectious agents, for example, but not always.[8]

As noted in chapter 19 on the role of the immune system and cancer risk, chronic inflammation can lead to cancer as it provides a ready-made mechanism that cancerous cells can use to their own advantage. Cancerous cells use the same proinflammatory cytokines and other molecules as the immune system does. But in this case, cancer deploys this system to promote the development of new blood vessels, boost cell division, and encourage damage to DNA through the release of radical oxygen species.

For a long time, researchers have suspected that chronic inflammation in the prostate can lead to prostate cancer. The results tend to be mixed, but prostate biopsy samples from radical prostatectomy (surgery to remove cancerous prostate gland) as well from benign prostatic hyperplasia often show inflammation. Some studies suggest that early prostate cancer cells may form in lesions usually linked to chronic inflammation.

Researchers have also noted that men who eat more fish and who use aspirin and other nonsteroidal anti-inflammatory drugs appear to have a lower risk for prostate cancer. As many types of fish are generous sources of omega-3 fatty acids, these beneficial fats may boost the production of proinflammatory cytokines, thus helping protect against prostate cancer by preventing inflammation. It's a paradox: while increased production of proinflammatory cytokines can help prevent inflammation, stimulating this production above a certain threshold can have an adverse effect and lead to chronic inflammation (for more, see chapter 19, "Immune System and Cancer Risk.").[4,7]

Sexually Transmitted Diseases

Having many sexual partners is associated with a raised risk for this cancer, probably because this behavior increases the chances of catching sexually transmitted diseases (STDs). However, it is not clear how an STD infection could lead to a higher risk for prostate cancer. It appears that the bacterial or viral agents in these diseases may promote chronic inflammation of prostate tissue, leaving the gland more vulnerable to cancer development. STDs may also play a role in prostate cancer because of the connection between these diseases and prostatitis. Some research points to human papillomavirus (types 16, 18, and 33) infection and HIV infection as possible higher prostate cancer risks; another study indicates that the STDs syphilis and recurrent gonorrhea are linked to an increased prostate cancer risk that is two or three times higher than the norm.

Note that no consistent link with any particular STD was found during large prospective studies of prostate cancer.[8]

Benign Prostatic Hyperplasia

One topic under investigation is whether an enlarged prostate can increase the risk for prostate cancer. An enlarged prostate, or a benign prostatic hyperplasia (BPH), occurs in the internal transition and periurethral zones, and prostate cancer generally develops in the gland's external, peripheral areas; thus BPH is not seen as a cancer risk—at least at present.

As older men are at high risk for—and often have—both enlarged prostates and prostate cancer, it can be difficult to determine any kind of independent function BPH may have in cancer development. Also, because so many older men have enlarged prostates, it is a challenge to rule this condition out in control groups. Yet the evidence is building for a pathogenic association between an enlarged prostate (BPH) and prostate cancer.[9]

SUMMARY

In spite of considerable research efforts, the causes of prostate cancer are not yet clearly understood. Scientists believe the disease is a result of a mix of genetic factors and environmental exposures. As this disease remains a major health threat, particularly for men in developed countries, all men should discuss prostate cancer screening with their doctors, particularly after age 50. It is important to note that the potential risk-reduction benefits of prostate cancer screening are controversial. This issue will be discussed further in chapter 20.

Chapter 15

Skin Cancer

About half of all known cancers are skin cancers. In fact, about one in five people in the United States will be diagnosed with skin cancer in their lifetime, according to the American Cancer Society.[16] Several types of skin cancer are known, although they are often classified as either melanoma skin cancer or nonmelanoma skin cancer. When skin cancer forms in the pigment-producing cells (melanocytes), it is called melanoma. Nonmelanoma skin cancer types include squamous cell carcinoma (appears on the squamous, or flat surface, cells of the skin) and basal cell carcinoma (grows on the round cells found under the squamous cells). Yet another type of nonmelanoma skin cancer is neuroendocrine carcinoma (or Merkel cell carcinoma), found in hormone-releasing skin cells.

Nonmelanoma skin cancers are the most common, diagnosed in more than 1 million people every year in the United States, with fewer than 1,000 dying from this disease annually. The mortality rate for melanoma skin cancer is much worse. While fewer people are diagnosed with this disease—an estimated 68,000 in the United States for 2010—the death toll adds up to nearly 9,000 annually.[1] This cancer has the most rapidly increasing incidence of malignancy. Melanoma causes 77 percent of skin cancer deaths, and in terms of years of life lost, it is also the second-most-deadly cancer after leukemia.[1] Since the 1970s, skin cancer survival rates have improved significantly, but no proven cure yet exists for the metastatic disease.

SYMPTOMS

Skin cancer usually is not painful in its early stages. The disease's most common early symptom is change: a different color or irregular border on a mole, a new growth or an alteration on an old growth, or a different texture such as the scaly rough skin in the precancerous condition actinic keratosis (a red and scaly growth; see below).

If cancer develops, more observable changes may take place: the shape or color of existing moles may alter, moles or growths may ooze or bleed, moles may itch or become unusually larger, and slow-to-heal sores may appear on a mole. Unexplained blood blisters may develop under toenails, or the edges of moles or growths may become irregular, jagged, and blurred.

It is important to note that it is normal for people to find new moles on their bodies now and then until they are into their 40s. The only cause for concern is when moles have an uneven color, irregular shape, or jagged edges. Some cases of actinic keratosis may not cause cancer, nor do most moles. Anyone with concerns about symptoms should consult a dermatologist for a diagnosis and for advice regarding sunscreen use.

TREATMENT

Surgery tends to be the first treatment option, as in the early stages, most squamous cell and basal cell skin cancers can be treated successfully. These cancers may even be completely removed during the biopsy. Other treatments that may be recommended include topical chemotherapy, photodynamic therapy, or radiation therapy. The treatment for melanoma depends on the stage of cancer and the age and health of the person diagnosed. Patients may have surgery, chemotherapy, or radiation treatments, among other therapies.

TYPES OF NONMELANOMA SKIN CANCER

Various types of skin cancer fall under the nonmelanoma category, including the very rare and second-most-fatal skin cancer, Merkel cell carcinoma.[3] The most common nonmelanoma skin cancers are basal cell carcinoma and squamous cell carcinoma.

Basal Cell Carcinomas

Basal cell carcinomas are named for where they begin: in the basal cell layer, the lowest layer of the epidermis. These typically appear on areas exposed to sunshine, such as the back of the neck or head. The incidence of this cancer reveals a change of habits: in the past, almost all the people diagnosed with this cancer were in their middle or senior years. Today this cancer is found in young people (the mean onset age is 25). A rare type of genetic basal cell skin cancer is Gorlin syndrome, also known as nevoid basal cell carcinoma syndrome. It is an autosomal dominant disorder, meaning that a person carrying only one mutated gene can be affected. This disease is characterized by basal cell carcinomas and appears in about 1 out of 60,000 cases. Gorlin syndrome appears equally in both genders and in all ethnicities.[12]

Unrelated patients with the same mutation for Gorlin syndrome can show different disease characteristics. Similarly, families with this syndrome and who have similar or identical mutations can differ dramatically in the expression of clinical features. This suggests that environmental exposures and genetics, alone or in combination, may influence Gorlin syndrome and how it manifests.

Most people with basal cell carcinoma will receive an optimistic prognosis. The cancer usually does not metastasize and so can often be cured with surgery. However, the cancer can be difficult to treat if it returns or if numerous cancerous lesions or tumors have appeared. Doctors may recommend cryosurgery or radiotherapy in some cases.[4,5]

While survival rates are encouraging, coping with the aftereffects of basal cell carcinoma may mean learning to live with scarring or damaged features. This is because the cancer attacks places most affected by sunshine—such as the face.

Squamous Cell Carcinomas

Squamous cell carcinomas are the most common type of human malignancy as they are found in up to 30 percent of all skin cancers. This disease tends to be more aggressive than basal skin cancers, frequently spreading to fatty tissues under the skin. This cancer is also more prone to invading lymph nodes and other areas across the body. Like basal cell carcinomas, squamous cell carcinomas develop on areas of the body that receive the most sunshine: the face, ears, back of neck, lips, and the backs of the hands—as well as in scars and skin ulcers. Squamous cell carcinomas occasionally take hold in the scaly, scabby bumps of actinic keratoses and infrequently in genital skin.

An early form of squamous cell carcinoma is Bowen disease, which appears as redder, more scaly and scabby patches than actinic keratoses. The risk factors include sun damage, as well as infection with human papillomavirus (HPV), the viral infection linked to genital warts and cervical cancer.[6]

Merkel Cell Carcinoma

Also called neuroendocrine carcinoma or trabecular cancer, Merkel cell carcinoma is a very rare and aggressive cancer that develops on or just below the surface of the skin, typically in sun-exposed areas. It's more commonly found in people with weak immune systems or in older people. It first appears as a painless, often flesh-toned or bluish-red lump on the skin and then grows rapidly and metastasizes at an early stage, so early detection is important. Although very uncommon, incidence of this cancer has tripled in the United States in the past

20 years (to about 1,500 cases annually). A 2008 study found evidence that the majority of cases of this cancer may be caused by a viral infection with what is now called the Merkel cell polyomavirus (MCV or MCPyV), found in 80 percent of Merkel cell carcinoma tumors.[15]

Melanoma Skin Cancer

Melanomas are dangerous; a person's chances of survival often depend on early detection and treatment. Although melanomas typically begin in moles or in what looks like healthy skin, in rare cases the cancer develops in the eyes, respiratory passageway, intestines, or brain.

The research shows that melanomas that develop on chronically sun-damaged skin are different from the melanomas that appear on skin without this damage. Melanomas that appear on skin with obvious long-term solar radiation exposure usually develop on older people and may accompany other sun-damage-related skin growths such as actinic keratoses. The association with keratoses suggests that the buildup of sun damage may be a prerequisite for this cancer.

Melanomas associated with less sun damage (or only occasional sun exposure) tend to appear on younger people marked by many moles and very few actinic keratoses. The key appears to be a genetic characteristic of the person's moles. Although, in general, genetic mutation is thought to play only a small role in melanoma development, melanomas that appear on skin that receives intermittent sun exposure tend to have more mutations of the tumor suppressor gene *BRAF* than other types of melanomas. Also, scientists have found that moles tend to show a high amount of *BRAF* mutations. This suggests that some who develop melanoma may have an increased susceptibility in their melanocytes to ultraviolet (UV) radiation and a higher probability of *BRAF* mutations—as well as more proliferation if those mutations happen. These people may be particularly vulnerable to UV exposure early in their lives.

It follows that people who do not have vulnerable melanocytes develop melanoma only after the cumulative damaging effects of repeated UV exposure. The mechanisms in this type of melanoma do not include *BRAF* mutations. These people with less susceptible skin are therefore more likely to have melanomas on areas that experience chronic sun damage, such as on their faces.[7,8]

RISK FACTORS

Although rarely seen in children, people of any age can develop skin cancer. Those most at risk for this disease are Caucasian men age 50 and older and with a low socioeconomic status, accounting for about half of all skin cancer deaths.

African Americans have much lower rates of skin cancer incidence, account-ing for about 0.9 cases per 100,000, although they are associated with greater morbidity.

Risk Factors for Nonmelanoma Skin Cancer

Sunlight, especially UV radiation, is considered a major risk factor for non-melanoma skin cancer and has a cumulative effect. This is why large amounts of solar radiation exposure can lead to skin cancer in people as young as age 20 or 30, although most people with the disease are in their senior years.

In particular, solar radiation exposure increases the nonmelanoma skin cancer risk for people who work outdoors (such as lifeguards) or who have fair skin, blue eyes, and light hair. A very small proportion of skin cancer cases are due to a genetic predisposition, such as Gorlin syndrome or xeroderma pigmentosum, a rare autosomal recessive genetic disorder of DNA repair mechanisms (the cancer, however, is prompted by sunshine). Patients taking immunosuppression drugs following organ transplantation or chemotherapy are at risk of getting nonmela-noma skin cancer.

A number of mutations in tumor suppressor genes (such as *BRAF, PTCH,* and *Pten*) are thought to increase the risk for skin cancer. Also, a mutation in the melancortin 1 receptor (*MC1R*) impedes melanin production, which raises the risk for skin cancer.[2]

Melanoma Risk Factors

Melanoma's relationship with solar radiation exposure is not clear. As described above, excess solar radiation exposure may promote some forms of melanomas, while genetic predisposition may lead to others. Factors such as altitude and skin pigmentation may be important in the risks for this cancer. For example, people who tan well are thought to have more protection; those living at higher altitudes may be at a higher risk.

Actinic Keratosis

Actinic (or solar) keratosis is a common skin disease that appears as reddened, scaly patches on the skin and is caused by long-term sun exposure. While these patches are not cancers, they are considered to be precancerous and some may de-velop into squamous cell carcinomas if left untreated. Actinic keratosis forms out of keratinocytes, the principal cell type in the outermost layer of skin. After years of harmful UV radiation exposure from the sun, these cells can become damaged and develop into lesions. These lesions can vary in size and color, and appear on skin most exposed to sunlight: the ears, face, back of the hands, and arms, for example, usually on people in their middle years or older and who have fair skin. These lesions typically appear in multiple and often do not cause any symptoms or signs other than the marks they make on the skin.

This skin disease can appear on anyone, but some people are more susceptible, particularly people with fair skin and light eyes who spend time outdoors. People with darker skin are less sensitive to solar UV radiation and so rarely develop this disease. As people age, they may be more at risk for actinic keratosis, as the condition grows slowly. Its early appearance is rare. Men appear to be at higher risk for this condition, although this may reflect that they are more likely to work outdoors and therefore experience more sun exposure.[9]

UV Radiation and Skin Cancer

The research shows that UV radiation exposure is a major risk factor for skin cancer, especially for nonmelanoma skin cancer. When skin is exposed to sunlight, it absorbs three different wavelengths of UV light: UVA, UVB, and UVC. The first two, UVA and UVB, have been demonstrated to cause DNA mutations and induce skin cancer in animal studies.[10]

Not all UVB radiation is bad for people, however. The body uses this type of light to make vitamin D, which can help prevent skin cancer. Scientists do not yet agree on how much sunshine is needed to make vitamin D without inducing skin cancer, however.

What Happens during Sun Exposure

Researchers believe that UV radiation exposure begins a chain of photochemical reactions that generate a photoprotective response or, possibly, skin damage. UV radiation stimulates keratinocytes, which eventually leads to melanin production (the brown pigment in skin), visible as a suntan. This coloring is a natural defense mechanism to prevent UV absorption.

If the solar radiation exposure is excessive or the melanin production mechanism is defective, UV radiation can induce the production of photoproducts (such as free radicals or ions) that harm DNA. Solar radiation can also break down water molecules to form radical oxygen species (ROS) in keratinocytes that eventually damage DNA. Sun damage may also lead to actinic keratosis, which in turn can develop into skin cancer.

Hereditary and Genetic Risk Factors

People with the rare genetic disorder xeroderma pigmentosum have a deficiency in their repair mechanisms for UV radiation damage. Some cases are so severe they must avoid all sunlight exposure, no matter how little, or risk developing skin cancer. Thus, people with this disease are susceptible to skin cancers early in their lives. Even in childhood, they may develop squamous and basal cell carcinomas and malignant melanomas. This predisposition to skin cancer is caused by mutations in several regulatory genes essential to DNA repair, leaving skin cells open to UV radiation's DNA-damaging effects. The strong connection between UV exposure and skin cancer in people with xeroderma pigmentosum is evidence for UV radiation as a key ingredient in skin cancer development.[9]

Research has shown that some skin cancer cells contain mutations in several genes, although the link between genetic mutation and skin cancer risk is generally believed to be low (few genetic defects have been found). UV radiation causes genetic mutations in the Patched gene, however, so this gene is thought to play a role in skin cancer. Other mutated genes found in skin cancer cells include *BRAF, CDKN2A, p53*, and *Pten*. The *BRAF* gene encodes for proteins that help control cell proliferation, and *BRAF* mutations are found in malignant melanomas. The *CDKN2A* gene (also known as *p*16) encodes a tumor suppressor protein that helps regulate the cell cycle. Mutations in this gene are a melanoma-susceptibility factor, found in half of all melanomas, making it the most commonly lost genomic region. The tumor suppressor genes *p*53 and *Pten* prevent the proliferation of cells with damaged DNA—an essential function in a healthy body. If these genes are mutated, cells with degenerate DNA may multiply.

The *p*53 gene also regulates programmed cell death (apoptosis), a necessary function that, in this case, eliminates skin cells with UV-induced damage—such as the dead skin that peels off after sunburn. Mutations in the *p*53 gene may mean the loss of this important function; a factor suspected to contribute to the initiation of skin cancer.[11]

PREVENTION: SUN AVOIDANCE AND SUNSCREEN

Some sunshine may be beneficial for most people. The human body needs UVB radiation to make vitamin D, which in turn helps prevent skin cancer and other health problems. Thus it seems a small amount of intermittent sun exposure may be helpful to human health—although it is still a matter of debate how much exposure is safe. Scientists do not know if the risk for skin cancer can be lowered by protecting skin from sunlight or other UV radiation sources such as sunlamps and tanning beds. Whether tanning beds and sunlamps pose the same risks as sunlight is still under debate.[13,14] It may be prudent to avoid the use of sunlamps and tanning beds in the meantime, particularly for young people.

Investigations on sunscreen's effectiveness against skin cancer have produced inconsistent data to date. Some research indicates a protective effect, while other research reports an increased skin cancer risk associated with sunscreen. The risks or benefits from sunscreen use may depend on individual skin pigmentation and the local climate, altitude, and geographic location. Only dermatologists can advise on sunscreen use.

SUMMARY

While all the causes of skin cancer are not yet known, laboratory studies on animals and cells have shown that prolonged exposure to solar UV radiation is a major risk factor for skin cancer. Other risk factors include prolonged exposure to artificial sunlight, light eyes and skin that burns easily, a weakened immune system, actinic keratosis, a history of bad sunburns, numerous moles, and a family history of melanoma. Caucasian men in their middle or senior years are most at risk. A person's risk for skin cancer may be further influenced by geographic latitude (and altitude) as well as ozone density.

Chapter 16

Occupation-Associated Cancer

It's a sad fact that many men and women have died because of on-the-job carcinogen exposure. People have known for some time that workplaces can be toxic. As mentioned in the introduction, as far back as 1775 an English physician connected the development of scrotal cancer in grown men to their childhood work as chimney sweeps. This is the earliest recorded association between cancer and an occupation-related carcinogen, and the first recorded instance of an environmentally influenced occupational cancer.[1] But it isn't the last.

Today, the research on occupation-related cancers continues, although it is usually conducted in developed countries. Some workplaces are clearly more associated with cancer risk than others. Studying these environments can help scientists investigate cancer's causes as well as the way the disease progresses, particularly if they find any unusual disease patterns in employees exposed to the same environmental toxins.

A complicating factor is time. Long periods of latency may pass after toxic exposures and it could be two or three decades before cancer appears. In spite of the challenges, researchers have managed to compile a growing list of recognized occupational and environmental carcinogens.

It appears that susceptibility to cancer may be related to environmental toxin exposure, especially those toxins encountered regularly in the workplace. Some of these toxic exposures may be obvious, such as the fumes from melting metals, but others are more subtle, such as microscopic asbestos particles, chemical fumes, or low levels of radiation exposure.

OCCUPATIONAL CARCINOGENS AND CANCER

Different workplace carcinogens can lead to different types of cancer: it seems most organs can be harmed by some kind of occupational toxin. For example, it's known that exposure to coal tar, benzidine, 2-naphthylamine, and 4-aminobiphenyle can promote bladder cancer.[5,6] Workers who are exposed to arsenic, beryllium, asbestos, bis(chloromethyl) ether, chromium, coal tar patch volatiles, radon, and silica are at higher risk for lung cancer.[8] Radium and asbestos exposure causes mesothelioma,[7] a rare cancer of internal organs' protective lining, while sulfuric acid mist can cause cancer of the larynx.[9] Liver cancer can be induced via encounters with arsenic, vinyl chloride, nickel, radium, and chromium,[10] while arsenic and coal tar can also promote skin cancer.[11] Lastly, benzene exposure is a risk factor for leukemia.[12] Furthermore, the risks for cancer climb higher when workers also smoke tobacco.

A LIST OF OCCUPATIONAL CARCINOGENS

Listing occupational carcinogens is useful in several ways. It helps establish safety regulations, provides a tool for cancer prevention, and can guide research priorities.

A partial summary of chemicals known to cause cancer in animals (but not adequately proved to cause cancer in humans) includes chlordecone, chloro-ortho-toluidine, dichloroethane, ethylhexyl phthalate, diethylhydrazine, ethyl acrylate, methylene dianiline, nitropropane, potassium bromate, safrole, styrene oxide, sulfallate, thioacetamide, toluene diisocyanate, and vinyl bromide.[2,3]

A LIST OF SUSPECTED CARCINOGENS

Several other substances found in workplaces are suspected to cause cancer, but more research is needed to assess their risk potential to humans. These substances include formaldehyde, which is used in construction materials such as the plywood, glues, installation materials, and coating products used to build homes and in the manufacture of industrial materials.

A short list of suspects includes the following:
Asbestos: a potential carcinogenic agent in gastrointestinal, kidney, and larynx cancers
Cadmium: may increase the risk for prostate cancer
Cutting oils: may raise the risk for gastrointestinal, lung, and skin cancers
Formaldehyde: may cause leukemia
Silica: associated with stomach cancer
Talc: suspected to promote lung and ovarian cancers
Vinyl chloride: associated with liver, brain, and ovarian cancer
Butadiene: thought to promote leukemia and lymphoma
Diesel fumes: linked to bladder and lung cancers
Dust: associated with stomach cancer
Some pesticides are potential risk factors for lymphatic and hematopoietic, lung, and prostate cancers.

While a few of these compounds are established carcinogens, including vinyl chloride and butadiene, others may contain toxic contaminants and polycyclic aromatic hydrocarbons (which are pre-carcinogens). When absorbed into the body, these compounds may then undergo chemical changes that transform them into carcinogens. A number of these occupational carcinogens may be found in the general environment or in medications, food, or other products. But because workplace conditions may mean employees are exposed for longer periods to these carcinogens, they may be at a higher risk for cancer than the average person. For example, men who had swept chimneys as boys in Victorian times were found to be at a greater risk for scrotal cancer than men who did not do this job in childhood. The chimney sweeps were exposed to the skin-irritating effects of carcinogenic polycyclic aromatic hydrocarbons found in soot.

While today it is known that the cancer-causing agents were the polycyclic aromatic hydrocarbons in soot, in some workplaces the causative agents for cancer are not as clear. Two examples of this are the higher incidence of lung cancer in painters and bladder cancer in people employed in the aluminum industry. It may be more understandable that people who work in places where they inhale diesel exhaust have a higher risk for lung cancer.[2]

ENVIRONMENTAL CARCINOGENS: INDOOR AND OUTDOOR AIR POLLUTANTS

People can be exposed to environmental carcinogens in various ways, through indoor and outdoor air pollutants and in contaminated soil and drinking water.

Several good-quality studies have looked into lung cancer risk from outdoor air pollution by measuring specific toxins. In general, the results have demonstrated that outdoor exposure to pollutants such as asbestos and radon increases the cancer risk.

As an example of an indoor environmental carcinogen, tobacco smoke is one of the more ubiquitous. It contains several known human carcinogens as well as other toxins and has been shown to cause lung cancer. Radon is another indoor air carcinogen and has been linked to lung cancer, as has wood smoke. Studies have shown that some Asian women face an increased risk of lung cancer when they cook and heat their homes with burning wood. Some people are unfortunate enough to have their drinking water contaminated with arsenic. This will increase their risk for bladder, skin, and lung cancers. The results, however, are inconclusive regarding the dangers of drinking water contaminated with chlorination by-products.

In total, about 29 established human carcinogens are found in workplaces. Another 30 substances are suspected carcinogenic agents, and at least 12 exposure circumstances involve exposure to carcinogens. This can make some occupations dangerous indeed. In fact, in spite of safety regulations, it is still common for people to be exposed to a variety of occupational carcinogens such as asbestos, coal tar, arsenic, and silica—particularly in developing countries.[4]

SUMMARY

Overall workplace safety improves as more researchers investigate occupational exposures. Unfortunately, as it often takes a couple of decades after a toxic exposure before cancer appears, most of the occupational carcinogens that have been identified to date are agents that workers were exposed to up to 30 years ago.

As new chemical and plastic manufacturing industries (among others) develop, it's likely that new, as yet unknown, occupational carcinogens are appearing as well. Carcinogenic agents may already be causing cancers that will be noticed 30 years down the road—or sooner.

Thanks to continuing research on human genetics, scientists may one day understand how genes and the environment interact to produce a disease in some, or all, cases. Researchers are particularly interested in learning what genes metabolize and excrete potential carcinogens, as well as what genes repair carcinogen-induced DNA damage.

A variety of scientific approaches may be helpful in raising the knowledge level in all areas. For example, new information on exposures may help pinpoint genes that are involved in the cancer process, which then may lead to discoveries regarding environmental factors. In the meantime, it's essential that safety regulations are upheld in workplaces to avoid exposing employees to occupational and environmental carcinogens—and putting them at risk for the misery of cancer.

Part II

Behaviors and Controversies

Chapter 17

Nutrition and Cancer

The concept that a well-balanced diet is essential to good health has been accepted for thousands of years. It was recognized by the father of Western medicine, Hippocrates (460–377 B.C.), who is credited for the following wisdom that is still relevant today: "If we could give every individual the right amount of nourishment and exercise, not too little and not too much, we would have found the safest way to health."[1]

In modern times, numerous studies have supported Hippocrates's theory on the therapeutic benefits of a balanced diet. The research has also shown that poor dietary choices can have unwelcome consequences. When a diet is out of balance, illness may ensue.

One well-known example of this is scurvy, a nutritional disorder that arises out of a lack of vitamin C, an essential nutrient found in vegetables and fruit. People with scurvy have weakened blood capillaries, and these bleed into tissues, including gums. Teeth become loose, and the person develops anemia. At one time, this disease was a serious problem for sailors and for people in places where fresh fruit and vegetables were not obtainable in winter months.

Even today, many people are eating diets deficient in essential nutrients—and perhaps eating too many harmful foods or foods prepared in ways that irritate the body. Several scientific studies estimate that up to 35 percent of all cancer deaths may be caused by unhealthy diets, with an additional 3 percent of deaths due to chronic alcoholism. The research is full of data linking dietary patterns with cancers of the breast, colon, liver, lung, and prostate. One prominent report suggests that a third of all cancer deaths could be avoided through dietary adjustments.

For dietary factors to have an impact in the long term, it may be that careful attention to nutrition beginning from childhood and adolescence is important. More research is needed to discover the relevant age when fruit and vegetables must be consumed to prevent cancer. All in all, however, scientific studies strongly support the consumption of fruit and vegetables to reduce cancer risk.[1,2]

An ideal diet contains fresh fruit and vegetables that are rich in phytochemicals—beneficial substances found in plants that can help protect against disease. For example, some vitamins with strong antioxidant properties defend tissues against carcinogen damage and keep the immune system strong so it can fight infection.

DIETARY FACTORS THAT HELP OR HARM

Phytochemicals

Phytochemicals (examples are vitamins C and E) help prevent cancer from developing by trapping (or scavenging) carcinogenic free radicals and by regulating key metabolizing enzymes known as phase I and phase II. The regulation of these enzymes is a major defense mechanism against foreign substances in the body.

Phase I drug-metabolizing enzymes (the cytochrome p450 family) make many carcinogenic products more water soluble so they can be excreted, while the phase II enzymes (for example, UDP-glucoronosyltransferases or glutathione S-transferases, such as GSTP1) catalyze the transformation of these foreign substances to assist their removal from the body's cells.[22]

It follows that if these key regulatory enzymes are inactivated because of genetic mutations, the risk for cancer increases. Scientists have often found mutations in the GSTP1 gene in prostate cancer cells. More on the function of phase I and phase II enzymes and how diet helps in their regulation is discussed later in this chapter.

Reactive Oxygen Species

Reactive oxygen species include carcinogens from harmful environmental exposures and by-products of the body's natural metabolic processes. As these can damage cell DNA and may cause cancer or promote the disease's development, one strategy in cancer prevention may be to find a way to block reactive oxygen species from inflicting damage on cellular DNA—perhaps through dietary intervention.

Dietary patterns vary around the world, and so does the cancer risk. The typical high-calorie, high-fat diet seen in the West is associated with a higher risk for cancer. Places where people tend to consume less fat and more fruit, vegetables, and whole grains show lower incidence of cancer. An example is the traditional Mediterranean diet, which features plenty of vegetables, legumes, fruit, nuts, mostly unrefined cereals, olive oil but little saturated fat, and fish. This diet typically has low amounts of dairy products (mostly as cheese and yogurt), modest amounts of meat or poultry, and small amounts of wine (usually) during meals. Several studies have shown the beneficial health effects of this way of eating.[3]

FACTORS THAT INCREASE CANCER RISK

The Food Source Counts

What we eat can contribute to cancer development. Any given food is a very complex substance that, along with nutrition, can deliver something harmful. For example, salmon is often celebrated as a health food as it is a rich source of omega-3 polyunsaturated fatty acids, a key component of a healthy diet. However, salmon are fatty carnivorous fish. Toxins and pollutants with DNA-damaging potential can build up in their flesh, and these can be passed on to people via the dinner plate.

This was a finding in one study that examined farmed and wild salmon stocks around the globe. The researchers discovered that in some places farmed salmon contained levels of polychlorinated biphenyls (PCBs) in amounts that, if eaten regularly, may increase consumers' cancer risk. That farmed salmon was found to have more contaminants than wild salmon raises another issue: that different sources of the same food may not offer the same benefits.[4]

Food Preparation Methods

Some ways of cooking can contribute to the cancer-causing substances in food. Charring meat or cooking meat at high temperatures transforms amino acids and proteins into carcinogens known as heterocyclic amines.[5] After metabolic activation (meaning they become active after enzymatic reactions) these carcinogens bind to DNA, producing what's called DNA adducts. These adducts damage the structure of DNA, or cause mutations, which then can lead to cancer.

Food Storage Issues

Some molds produce toxins called genotoxins when they contaminate food. The fungus aflatoxin B is a common peanut contaminant, while fumonisin B is known to contaminate corn (for more, see chapter 6, "Esophageal Cancer." These genotoxic agents appear as microconstituents in food and can behave as dietary carcinogens.

A Lack of Key Nutrients

A lack of key nutrients may increase cancer risk. Recent research suggests that the body's folate (a B vitamin) levels have an effect on colorectal cancer. Folate plays a role in metabolic reactions and is a critical coenzyme for DNA synthesis and methylation. A lack of folate may mean these essential functions are not performed properly, possibly contributing to tumor development.[6]

Excessive Fat Consumption

Eating too much fat, particularly from animals, can lead to obesity and a higher cancer risk.[7] A risk factor for several cancer diseases, obesity may lead to cancer in a number of ways. Obese people often have acid reflux, a condition that irritates and damages the esophageal epithelium and may promote the development of adenocarcinoma (cancer of the epithelia, originating in glandular cells). People with obesity also have large amounts of stored fat in their adipose (fat) cells. Having surplus fat cells may stimulate the body to make too much estrogen and androgen hormones. This may explain why high-fat diets are associated with breast, ovarian, and prostate cancer risk.

GENETIC MUTATIONS AND DIET

Some people seem to make all sorts of unhealthy choices, such as eating too much, eating the wrong foods, drinking excessively, and smoking, yet they still live long healthy lives without cancer. Credit genetics. Small genetic differences can determine a person's metabolic activity, in beneficial ways or not. This can moderate the level of cancer risk, in spite of harmful habits. Catalyzed by enzymes, these metabolic reactions vary between people, usually because of small mutations. These may be single nucleotide polymorphisms (SNPs), or changes in the genes that encode enzymes. Mutations such as these can be common to families, ethnic groups, or unique to one person and can affect how substances in the diet influence health. The difference between various ethnic groups regarding cancer rates and mortality may be related to the number of SNPs common to each population.

Of course, some of these mutations can be harmful, as can be seen from a variation in the *MTHFR* gene. This gene makes an enzyme (called methylenetetrahydrofolate reductase) that transforms homocysteine (an amino acid) into methionine, an essential amino acid needed in DNA synthesis. Mutations in the *MTHFR* gene can mean weaker enzyme activity and therefore less processing of homocysteine into methionine. DNA damage may follow, raising the risk for cancer if people with this mutation also have a folate deficiency.

Studies have shown that people who eat plenty of folate-rich foods tend to have a reduced risk for colorectal neoplasia, or abnormal colorectal tissue masses. Folate is essential for the synthesis of nucleotides, the molecules that make up DNA and RNA and are involved in metabolism, and for the provision of methyl groups (important biochemical structures) during chemical reactions. Recent research on genetic mutations in folate-metabolizing enzymes suggests these altered enzymes may induce or help induce colorectal cancer. Therefore, it is possible the connection between folate and cancer has to do with an altered form of *S*-adenosyl-methionine for methylation reactions (including DNA methylation) and fewer key nucleotides processed for DNA synthesis and repair.[8]

Another mutated gene can have a negative impact on the health of red meat eaters who like their steak or burgers cooked at high temperatures and even charred. Some people have a rapid variant (a fast acetylator) of the enzyme (*N*-acetyltransferase) that metabolizes carcinogenic heterocyclic amines, and some have a slow-variant mutation. Those with the rapid variant have an increased risk for colon cancer when they eat a lot of red meat compared to those with the slow variant. Thus, a person's colon cancer risk with respect to red meat consumption depends on two factors: the person's genotype and the carcinogens he or she is exposed to because of cooking methods.[9]

FOODS TO HELP REDUCE CANCER RISK

Although people have genetic differences that affect their metabolic activities and their susceptibility to cancer, numerous studies support the theory that eating fruit and vegetables can help reduce cancer risk. The epidemiological research strongly indicates that eating generous amounts of particular fruit and vegetables lowers the risk of several cancers, including colorectal, esophageal, stomach, and lung cancers. For example, the *Allium* genus vegetables (onions, leeks, garlic, chives, and shallots) contain flavonols and organosulfur (organic compounds that contain sulfur) and other bioactive compounds that may be anticarcinogenic, according to animal and test tube studies. A long list of bioactive components in food have been found to protect the body from cancer (at least in animal model systems). These include essential nutrients such as vitamins C, D, and E and calcium, selenium, folate, and zinc. Also on the list are several nonessential food components, such as carotenoids, indoles, allyl sulfur compounds, flavonoids, conjugated linoleic acid, and omega-3 fatty acids.[10]

The following section focuses on the bioactive components of well-known fruit and vegetables and their potential benefits as anticancer agents.

Tomatoes

Tasty and versatile, the tomato is also a nutritional powerhouse and potential anticancer agent. Many epidemiological studies indicate that a diet rich in tomatoes and tomato products may help reduce the risk for prostate cancer, thanks (in part) to lycopene, a phytochemical and the food's primary red carotenoid. (Lycopene amounts vary by tomato type—some yellow varieties may not have any, although these contain other valuable nutrients such as vitamin C.)

While fresh watermelon and pink grapefruit also contain lycopene, sources show that up to 85 percent of the lycopene in most people's diets comes from tomato products, such as canned tomato sauce or paste.[11] Tomatoes contain potassium, folate, and other carotenoids and phytochemicals, including the suspected anticancer agents polyphenols. Tomatoes are generously endowed with flavonols; close to 98 percent of the flavonols in the tomato skin are conjugated forms of quercetin and kaempferol, which have antioxidant properties. Tomatoes also contain small amounts of naringenin (a flavanone, a type of flavonoid) in its conjugated form.

Along with those benefits, tomatoes are rich in vitamins A, C, and E. When compared to other popular vegetables, only carrots can offer more vitamin A than tomato-based foods. Tomato products, especially tomato paste, are also high in fiber, another factor thought to lower the risk for cancer.

These nutrients and phytochemicals often have antioxidant properties and, acting with lycopene, may increase the benefits of eating tomatoes.[11,12]

THE POTENTIAL ACTIONS OF TOMATO PHYTOCHEMICALS

Lycopene may offer its benefits in several ways. Scientific studies suggest the phytochemical behaves as an antioxidant and regulates cell-cycle progression.[27] Lycopene and other tomato phytochemicals may also regulate hormone and growth factor signaling in prostate cells, one possible explanation for tomato's suspected anticancer actions. For example, large amounts of free-circulating insulin-like growth factor (a protein that sparks cell proliferation and cell-death resistance) in the blood are linked with increased cancer risks. Case-control studies have examined changes in the activity of this protein. In general, studies show that eating cooked tomatoes can decrease serum insulin-like growth factor-1 levels. In one study, rats given lycopene supplementation had significantly lower levels of insulin-like growth factor-1 (although whole tomatoes may be more effective than lycopene supplements; see below).

A population-based study showed a strong tendency for lower serum insulin-like growth factor-1 and higher insulin-like growth factor binding protein-3 (which prevents stimulation of cell proliferation) after subjects ate more ketchup and drank more tomato juice.

The lower ratio of insulin-like growth factor-1 to insulin-like growth factor binding protein-3 is thought to be beneficial. This is because the binding protein helps stop the growth factor from promoting cell multiplication, which could lead to cancer.

Studies show that tomato polyphenols (quercetin, kaempferol, and rutin) and lycopene can stop insulin-like growth factor-1 signaling in vitro, thereby preventing cell proliferation. Because of the phytochemical complexity within the simple tomato, it may be that whole tomato products are more effective in inhibiting cancer development than supplementation with pure lycopene.[11]

Garlic

Garlic (*Allium sativum* L.) is valued around the world for its culinary uses as well as its medicinal properties. Garlic has been long regarded as a strong preventive medicine as well as a therapeutic medical agent in India, China, and ancient Egypt. Recent research has shown the bulb's pharmacological effects, including its antifungal, antibacterial, antithrombotic (reduces clotting), antioxidant, and anticancer properties. Several epidemiological and laboratory investigations have shown an inverse relationship between garlic consumption and death by colorectal and stomach cancers.[13]

Garlic has several demonstrated actions that are very beneficial to people. First of all, the bulb's antioxidants help remove oxygen free radicals that can accumulate as metabolic by-products of carcinogens. Next, research on a major compound in garlic, ajoene, has shown that this compound can induce cell death in malignant cells in people with leukemia. Similarly, studies have shown garlic's allicin compound can impede the multiplication of breast, endometrial, and colon cancer cells in vitro (via test tube or petri dish).[12]

The research continues on how garlic acts to prevent gastric cancer. One clue is the herb's antibacterial qualities, which act against invaders such as *H. pylori,* credited in part to garlic's thiosulfinate concentration. Recently, researchers found that garlic clove extract (standardized for its thiosulfinate concentration) prevented *H. pylori* growth. The components responsible for garlic's odor and flavor, organosulfur compounds, may offer more general anticancer effects. Flavanols are also plentiful in garlic, especially kaempferol, and these can help detoxify carcinogens. One researcher showed that garlic powder could defend the body against induced mammary epithelial cell DNA adduct formation.[13]

Garlic's antimicrobial ability is significant. Research demonstrated that garlic extract's bactericidal effect killed 93 percent of *Staphylococcus epidermidis* and *Salmonella typhi* within three hours. Yeasts were eradicated within one hour by the garlic extract. (The spice clove showed the next strongest bactericidal effect in the study and killed yeasts within five hours of contact.) As bacteria that now show resistance to some antibiotics are sensitive to garlic, this herb has great potential as an antimicrobial agent.[14]

Cruciferous Vegetables

Broccoli, cauliflower, cabbage, watercress, and Brussels sprouts: a powerful category of phytochemical-rich vegetables that may lower the risk for a variety of cancers, according to epidemiological data. Cruciferous vegetables alone contain isothiocyanates, a nutrient credited with the category's anticarcinogenic effects.

Studies using animal models have shown that isothiocyanates can defend against cancer induced by toxins such as tobacco smoke carcinogens. Several naturally occurring isothiocyanates were shown to impede carcinogen-induced tumor growth and development in animal models. In addition, a high consumption of cruciferous vegetables was linked with a reduced risk of a variety of cancers in case-controlled epidemiological studies.[15]

The isothiocyanates in cruciferous vegetables do their magic by helping eliminate carcinogens from the body during the metabolic process, thus offering anticancer benefits. Nearly all carcinogens taken into the body, whether they come from the diet or the environment, must be metabolized, an enzymatic process that happens in two phases. In phase I, carcinogens are oxidized and subjected to reduction and hydrolysis to make the toxic molecules water soluble. The family of enzymes that process carcinogens through phase I are the cytochrome p450 enzymes.

As a result of the enzymatic action in phase I, the procarcinogens (those that become carcinogenic only after being metabolized) are typically transformed into highly reactive intermediates that can bind to and cause problems for DNA, RNA, and protein. Next up, the phase II enzymes further process the reactive intermediates with other factors in the body, making the toxins even more water soluble for easy waste disposal (through bile or urine). A considerable amount of scientific data shows that the anticancer action of isothiocyanates may be in assisting phase II enzymatic action and in binding to phase I components and inhibiting their action or by working as a competitive inhibitor.[16]

Green Tea

Green tea is one of the most popular drinks in the world and also one of the most studied. Much scholarly interest has focused on the polyphenols in tea thanks to their potent antioxidant activity. In fact, tea drinks have shown an ability to impede cancer development. Consequently, people who regularly sip this beverage have a lower risk for a variety of cancers such as gastric and colorectal cancer. Although black and oolong teas also offer similar health benefits (they are from the same plant as green tea, but are processed differently), green tea has been found to have higher antioxidant potency.

Green tea benefits the human body in a number of different ways. The antioxidant action of its polyphenols soaks up and deactivates free radicals, and its polyphenols have been shown (along with those of black tea's) to impede or prevent cancer formation in breast tissue by *in vitro* (in test tube) and *in vivo* (in live animals) studies. One of the main polyphenols of green tea, epigallocatechin gallate, has an action that may prevent tumor growth: it stops telomerase activity.

This process occurs via an undiscovered mechanism. Impeding telomerase activity slows down cell proliferation; in one study, this was shown to shrink tumors in laboratory mice.[17]

Soy

Numerous studies show dietary soy's anticancer action on breast tumors. Of particular interest among some researchers is the soy isoflavone genistein. Along with other soy phytochemicals, genistein has been shown to prevent the growth of tumors after implantation of MCF-7 breast cancer cells (a commercially available breast cancer cell line used in research) in studies using in vitro and in vivo methods. This suggests that genistein can prevent estrogen-dependent MCF-7 tumors in animals. More study is needed to know if it can prevent tumors in people.

The health of Asian women offers more support for the benefits of green tea and soy foods—both major constituents of the Asian diet. Asian women have a much lower incidence of breast cancer, possibly as a result of these foods.[23,24,25] The anticancer activity of these foods may be enhanced when they are taken together. One study showed that mixing tea components with soy phytochemicals created possible synergistic qualities in limiting growth of estrogen-dependent breast tumors in human subjects.[18] It is possible these anticancer benefits of soy may result only from long-term and frequent soy consumption.

Research has shown that soy foods can prevent not only breast cancer but also cancers of the colon and prostate. Research on soy foods and prostate cancer risk showed that men who ate soy products decreased their risk for prostate cancer by nearly 30 percent. The protective factor may be due to soy's high levels of phytoestrogens and could explain why Asian men in their countries of origin have a low rate of prostate cancer.[19]

It's important to note that soy's anticancer benefits with respect to breast cancer are controversial because of the food's high levels of phytoestrogens. A concern is that phytoestrogens could contribute to breast cancer risk in some cases. This topic is discussed in chapter 20.

Vitamin D

Whether synthesized from sunlight's ultraviolet (UV) B rays or taken as a supplement, adequate vitamin D is essential to good health. Its main job is to ensure healthy bones by upholding levels of calcium and phosphorus in the blood. The vitamin also helps promote bone mineralization.

First, however, vitamin D (from supplement or sunlight synthesis) must be converted in the kidney and liver to its active form, 1,25 dihydroxyvitamin D. It then acts as a hormone and signals the intestines to absorb more phosphorus and calcium. Thus, a lack of vitamin D can mean not enough calcium and phosphorus are absorbed, resulting in frail and thin bones. A serious deficiency could lead to weak bone-related illnesses such as rickets in children or osteomalacia in adults.

But recent research has shown that this vitamin may also play other key roles: assisting the immune system and helping regulate cell growth and differentiation. Vitamin D may also offer protection against various cancers, according to epidemiological, laboratory, and animal studies. One conclusion is that people may decrease their risk for cancer by increasing the amount of vitamin D and calcium in their diets or by allowing the body to make more vitamin D from sunlight.

Sunlight exposure is perhaps the most important source of vitamin D to most people around the world. Specifically, the sun's UVB rays are needed to activate vitamin D synthesis in the body. Various factors, however, can inhibit this process. UV exposure and therefore natural vitamin D synthesis can be limited by cloud cover, smog, sunscreen, geographic latitude, time of day, and the seasons. For example, people living in Boston, Massachusetts, from November through February will likely not receive enough sunlight exposure to produce needed vitamin D levels in their skin.

While complete cloud cover lowers UV exposure by half, shade reduces the exposure by 60 percent—even more when the air is full of industrial pollution. Pollution may be a contributing factor in cases of rickets in some places in the world where dietary levels of vitamin D are low.

We know excess solar UV radiation exposure is linked to skin cancer (see chapter 15, "Skin Cancer"), but how much sunshine is sufficient to ensure maximum safety and benefits? Some data suggest a daily, brief 10- to 15-minute exposure is enough time for adequate vitamin D synthesis.[28]

The use of sunscreen has become somewhat controversial. Studies examining the benefits of sunscreen have mixed results: some studies show sunscreen protects skin, while other studies indicate that the use of sunscreen is associated with a higher risk for skin cancer. A disadvantage to sunscreen use is that a sun protection factor (SPF) of eight or higher will block the UV rays needed to make vitamin D.

In general, although people are still recommended to use sunscreen to help prevent skin cancer and sunburn, a better approach may be to limit sun exposure to 10 or 15 minutes (before sunscreen use) to allow for adequate vitamin D synthesis. One final note regarding vitamin D: people with limited sun exposure should ensure they have good sources of vitamin D in their diets.

Selenium

Meat, bread, nuts, and plant-based foods are common sources of the essential mineral selenium. In the body, selenium combines with proteins to produce key antioxidant enzymes called selenoproteins. These enzymes help prevent free radicals from damaging cells and ultimately contributing to chronic disease such as heart disease and cancer. Selenoproteins also support the immune system and help moderate thyroid function. Selenium may also stop or slow tumor growth by improving immune cell activity and suppressing the extension of blood vessels into tumors.[26]

Although selenium is necessary for good health, the human body needs this mineral only in trace amounts. Yet even tiny amounts can be hard to come by, in some places. As most people around the world get their dietary selenium through plant foods, the amount of selenium in various vegetables will depend on the mineral's availability in the soil where the food is grown. This can vary greatly.

Research has shown that the soil in the high plains of North and South Dakotas and northern Nebraska is rich in selenium.[29] People living in those areas tend to have some of the highest selenium intakes in the United States, although food distribution patterns in the United States tend to ensure the population receives selenium in their diets, even those in low-selenium geographic areas. Animals grazing or eating grains from selenium-rich soil also have higher muscle levels of selenium. In China and Russia, however, some soils have very little selenium. As people in those regions tend to eat locally grown foods, selenium deficiency becomes a problem.

People with higher blood levels of selenium (because of higher intake of selenium) appear to have a reduced risk of death from several cancer diseases, such as colorectal, lung, and prostate cancers, according to observational studies (in which people are observed and outcomes are studied).[30] It's interesting to note that in the United States, incidence of nonmelanoma skin cancer is much higher in areas with little selenium in the soil.

Vitamin E

Many studies have pointed to vitamin E as a potent antioxidant and tumor-growth inhibitor. Researchers found that vitamin E impedes, or slows, the growth of prostate cancer cells in vitro and that the anticancer effects are enhanced when combined with selenium (and possibly other antioxidants).[20] Dietary sources abound for vitamin E, including nuts, seeds, and vegetable oils, as well as fortified cereals and leafy green vegetables.

SUMMARY

How food can affect our cancer risk is an ongoing topic of intense research. The current literature contains many inconsistencies, however, probably because of the multiple factors that determine how food components—such as phytochemicals—affect people. These factors include variations in how food components can find or act on key targets, genetic mutations affecting absorption of dietary components as well as their metabolism or site of action, or mutations in enzyme DNA methylation patterns. All of these factors can affect the body's response to beneficial food components and vice versa. Also, food component variation may increase or reduce gene expression differently in people, a possible explanation for inconsistencies.

To have a positive impact on key cancer-prevention processes, bioactive food components (such as vitamins or polyphenols) need to be available in the right amounts at the target sites. They also have to be in the correct metabolic form (via enzyme processing).

Future research and study in this area of molecular nutrition promises to offer a much more thorough understanding of how food components can affect cancer risk. One day it may even be possible to design diets specific to individuals to reduce their risk for cancer—and stop tumor growth.[21]

Chapter 18

Body Weight and Cancer

Second only to tobacco smoke, obesity is a leading cause of premature yet preventable death in the United States. The number of obese people in this country has more than doubled in the past 25 years—and that includes children. Obesity rates are especially high in African Americans, Hispanics, and people of low socioeconomic status.

But while the United States appears to lead this trend, obesity is now becoming a global epidemic. The potential impact on the health of people around the world is staggering. Evidence from scientific and epidemiological studies indicates that being overweight or obese raises the chances for several diseases and conditions, including heart disease, stroke, and high blood pressure and cancers of the prostate, colon, esophagus, endometrium, and breast (in postmenopausal women).[1]

Fundamentally, the process seems simple: habitually consuming too many calories leads to chronic weight gain and, if unchecked, to obesity.

There appear to be at least two main schools of thought regarding obesity. One is false: that some people have no self-control over what they eat and will not get off the couch to exercise, and so they are slothful, gluttonous, or both. This false belief leads to discrimination of overweight or obese people regarding their body size, whether on the job, in the mall, at school, or anywhere the general public meets. The scientific community, however, knows obesity is a much more complicated problem that is connected to contemporary life and the environment in which we live. Changes over the past few decades in the physical and social environment have meant a readier availability of high-calorie foods, while sedentary habits have become much more common because of the demands of urban life and working conditions. This becomes more evident as populations move from rural lifestyles to a citified way of life and, often, less physical activity. Another important factor is that obese people may also have genetic predispositions that promote weight gain.

ENERGY BALANCE

The expression "energy balance" refers to the intersection of food consumption, physical activity, and genetic makeup—the balance between energy consumption and energy output. Scientists use this concept to consider the resulting consequences and possible cancer risk when one factor outweighs the rest.

A positive energy balance means increased fat mass (adiposity), while a negative balance indicates weight loss. A stable body weight indicates a balance.

"Energy intake" is your diet, measured in calories, but energy can be expended (or spent) in three ways: through physical exercise or activity; the basal, or resting, metabolic rate; and the thermal effect of digesting food.[2] While it's not exercise, the body's processing of food (through digestion, absorption, and metabolism) requires a significant amount of energy, although this will also depend on the type of food eaten. Dietary fat, for example, is quickly transformed into body fat, while carbohydrates take more energy to process. The basal metabolic rate, meanwhile, needs energy to preserve normal body functions such as circulation, respiration, endocrine secretion, kidney filtration, and excretion. The energy expended through physical exercise can be increased or decreased at will, but the energy spent by the human body's metabolic and digestive systems is subject to genetics, endocrine responses, metabolism, and physical activity.

The notion of energy balance helps scientists investigate the origins of a variety of chronic diseases known to be linked to obesity, such as cancer.

It stands to reason that obese people have an abnormally high and unhealthy proportion of body fat. For a precise measure of a person's proportion of body fat, scientists and health professionals frequently turn to body mass index (BMI). BMI is the ratio of weight to height: a person's weight in kilograms (Kg) divided by a person's height in meters, multiplied by itself.

BMI offers a more accurate measure of body fat than weight alone because it adjusts for height. The healthy range of BMI is from 18.5 to 24.9. Someone with a BMI lower than 18.5 is deemed underweight, while a person with a BMI higher than 25 is considered overweight. A person with a BMI over 30 is thought to be obese.

Recent surveys showed that nearly two-thirds of U.S. adults have a BMI higher than 25, indicating they are overweight, while nearly one-third of all Americans are obese. As rates for childhood obesity are also rising, rates for adult obesity in the future will also continue to increase, along with obesity-related cancers and other chronic diseases such as diabetes and heart disease.[3]

Body Weight Maintenance

The human body maintains a stable body weight through a process known as energy homeostasis. This involves a series of biochemical actions to keep a steady supply of energy stored in body fat. These biochemical actions can be described as three mechanisms: afferent signals, efferent signals, and central processing. Afferent signals are usually hormones such as insulin (from the pancreas), gherlin (from the stomach), or leptin (from fat tissue) that are sent to central processing in the hypothalamus to report on the body's energy state. The hypothalamus then signals the efferent system to either boost appetite when the body needs food or to stop eating and get moving—all to restore energy balance and baseline body weight.

To maintain homeostasis, these mechanisms must be precisely regulated. A number of researchers have put forth various theories on how this might be done. One scientist proposed in 1953 that the body produces inhibitory signals in proportion to its stored body fat to limit food consumption, when needed. This means that if a person experienced weight loss or starvation, these inhibitory signals would be reduced until increased appetite helped correct the energy deficit (in lost body fat).[4] But this explanation does not cover how appetite and food consumption are controlled during meals. A proposal in 1973, however, pointed to the onset of satiety as the major determinant of how much is eaten at a meal. In general, people experience satiety after their brains receive hormonal signals (called satiety factors), such as proteins released from the gastrointestinal tract, that inhibit appetite or hunger.[5]

More recently, in 2000, a scientific team proposed a unified model based on the previous two hypotheses. They suggested that changes in the leptin and insulin concentrations are tied to compensatory adjustments of food consumption. Thus, low blood levels of leptin and insulin that occur during times of food scarcity stimulate the desire to eat and depress energy expenditure. At times of plenty, high levels of leptin and insulin suppress appetite after interacting with satiety circuits to limit food consumption and restore energy balance.[6] More on how leptin and insulin cooperate to regulate energy balance is described below.

Hormones and Body Weight

The notion of long-term energy balance regulation has changed dramatically since the discovery of the hormone leptin, found in white adipose (fat) tissue. Some studies show an association between energy balance regulation and glucose (simple sugar) metabolism.

The current working hypothesis on energy balance suggests leptin and insulin hormones are critical to homeostasis regulation. Leptin (from fat cells) and insulin (from the pancreas) are secreted into blood concentrations proportionate to body fat mass. These hormones enter the brain and the hypothalamus, bind to their target neurons, and activate their receptors. These pathways balance energy consumed versus energy expended, which in turn determines the amount of body fuel stored as fat.

A number of mechanisms function behind the scenes in regard to insulin, leptin, and body fat. As body fat accumulates, more insulin is released, leading to higher amounts of insulin traveling to the brain. This should help stop further weight gain. But the body also needs insulin to convert various foods such as sugars into energy, however; and when pancreatic cells cannot increase insulin secretion to meet the body's needs, hyperglycemia (excessive blood sugar) develops. This likely contributes to the link between obesity and type 2 diabetes.

The leptin-secretion mechanism is different. It appears this hormone is limited when the body's levels of total fat are low, such as during long-term fasting, malnutrition, and calorie-restriction diets. Studies have shown food deprivation reduces plasma leptin concentrations in humans and rodents, which may be linked to lower body fat.[20] Leptin levels do not remain low, however, once food intake increases—nor does body fat content. In other words, leptin appears to be a hormone that works to suppress appetite. Research suggests that blood serum leptin levels indicate metabolic energy output and that high serum leptin levels are seen in people with breast, colon, endometrial, and prostate cancers.[21]

Higher leptin levels are linked to an increased risk of bigger and more dangerous tumors, although it is not clear why. It may be that high leptin levels mean more fat cells, which in turn spark the release of estrogen and androgen, which speed hormone-dependent cancer cell proliferation. Leptin may also have a role in several inflammatory mechanisms that contribute to obesity-related diseases by behaving as a proinflammatory cytokine.[7,8] This suggests high leptin levels promote cancer development.

Age-Related Weight Gain

Clearly, the hormone mechanisms discussed above are simplistic models. The ease with which some people put on excess weight seems contrary to the proposition that food consumption is a highly regulated process.

A number of variables that are biologically unregulated can affect how much food people eat. These variables are social factors, time of day, convenience, cost, and emotional state, among other issues that cause food consumption to change on a daily and an individual basis. In most people, however, their cumulative food intake matches their energy expenditure quite well when measured over time and many meals.

Yet with age comes a decline in body muscle mass and, consequently, a decline in metabolism. After age 45, the average person loses about 10 percent of his or her muscle mass every 10 years. This may mean losing from a third to a half pound of muscle annually—and gaining that same amount in body fat. This has a strong impact on metabolism as muscle mass burns more calories than fat. The key point is that as people get older, they need fewer calories to maintain the same body weight. As regular exercise (which helps counter this effect) can become difficult for older people, it is common for people to gain weight as they age.

Genetic Predisposition

Scientists have found several genetic mutations that influence food consumption in severely obese mice. These mutations occur on key appetite-signaling pathways. As the mouse genome shares high DNA sequence identity with the human genome, many of the mutated genes linked to obesity in mice are also associated with obesity in people. For example, defective leptin signaling causes obesity in mice and people.[9]

But most people who struggle with obesity do not have irregularities in leptin or its receptor; they appear to have leptin resistance (their bodies appear to be unresponsive to leptin). This could be a result of other defects, possibly in mediators such as agouti-related protein (increases appetite and decreases metabolism) and its receptor, the melanocortin-4 receptor.

Genetic predisposition likely causes less than 10 percent of human obesity. This disease, therefore, must be a consequence of a complicated interaction of environmental factors such as an increased availability of high-calorie food, a lower need for physical activity, and a predisposition to genetic abnormalities in the energy balance pathway.[10]

Obesity's Socioeconomic Link

In the United States, people with the highest poverty rates and the least education also tend to have the highest rates of obesity, possibly because of the low cost of high-calorie (energy-dense) foods. Unfortunately, an inverse relationship exists between food's energy density (measured as energy per unit weight, or kilocalories per gram) and energy cost (dollars per kilocalorie). The result is that diets featuring fresh vegetables, fruit, nuts, and lean meats and fish are much more expensive than diets full of refined flours, sugar, salt, and added fats. Anyone trying to reduce a grocery budget may find the daily calorie count climbing—and his or her waistline measurements. Prepackaged and prepared foods may be convenient, but these foods often have more added sugar, salt, and fat and so increase the risk for weight gain.[11]

Fat Deposits and Cancer: Location Counts

All body fat is not equal. Fat wrapped around the middle of the body (abdominal fat) appears to pose a greater health risk than fat that accumulates on the hips, buttocks, or elsewhere, as it is more metabolically active (abdominal fat cells seem to be more prone to inducing insulin resistance than fats stored elsewhere on the body).

Exercise may be the way to better health for people with excessive abdominal fat. Although reducing the number of calories eaten also helps people lose weight, some studies have shown that exercise preferentially reduces intra-abdominal fat. People who develop regular exercise habits are also more likely to maintain a healthy weight after losing excess fat.[12]

Cancer Diseases Linked to Higher BMI

Plenty of research shows a strong link between obesity and cancer. Epidemiological studies demonstrate that men and women with a BMI of more than 30 significantly increase their risks for death from a variety of cancers. These diseases include colorectal, esophageal, non-Hodgkin lymphoma, gallbladder, kidney, multiple myeloma, and pancreatic cancers.

Men with higher BMI also have a higher risk for prostate and stomach cancer, while women with a higher BMI have a raised risk for death by breast, cervical, ovarian, and uterine cancers.[1] (However, some studies have found that the increase in breast cancer linked to obesity is only in women who do not take hormone replacement therapy.)

Obesity and Breast Cancer

The timing counts, too, regarding weight gain and cancer risk. Some studies show that women boost their breast cancer risk if they put on extra weight after age 18, especially after menopause, but they may lower their breast cancer risk if they lose excess body fat after menopause. Thus it may be that some women can avoid breast cancer by losing weight after menopause.[13] (Note that the current evidence supports the loss of excess weight at any stage as a way to reduce cancer risk.)

Each woman's menopausal status is a key to how obesity will affect her breast cancer risk. Young obese women have less of a risk for breast cancer than do healthy-weight women, although this advantage disappears after menopause. At that point, obese women have a one-and-a-half times higher risk for death from breast cancer than do women with a healthy weight. This suggests that about 10,000 U.S. women every year could avoid death from breast cancer by keeping a healthy body weight (a BMI under 25). It is important to note that the increased risk of breast cancer linked to obesity has been found only in women who do not take hormone replacement therapy. This indicates that hormones play a role when obese or overweight women develop breast cancer.

The higher risk of breast cancer for obese women after menopause appears to be caused by the estrogen-generating qualities of fat (adipose tissue). The ovaries produce most of the estrogen in the female body until menopause, when their function declines. At this time, fat tissue becomes the body's main estrogen source. As heavy women have more fat tissue, their bodies often have estrogen levels that are 50 to 100 percent higher than those of healthy-weight women. More estrogen circulating in the body means more enhanced cell growth and proliferation, especially in estrogen-sensitive tissues. This can promote breast cancer development.

Some of the cancer risk may depend on the location of women's body fat. As mentioned earlier, abdominal fat is riskier than fat that rests on hips, buttocks, or thighs. This may be because abdominal fat is connected to insulin resistance, which leads to an increase in growth factor expression and enhanced tumor growth. Obesity creates another breast cancer risk for women by increasing the density of breast tissue. It is much more difficult to find early-stage breast cancer tumors in breasts with dense tissue mass.

Regardless of menopausal status, women who are obese appear to have an increased risk for endometrial cancer, possibly up to a four times greater risk than women of healthy weight.[14] All in all, epidemiological studies suggest that obese women are more likely to die from breast cancer than women of healthy weight.

Obesity and Colon Cancer

People who are obese are more likely to develop colon cancer than people who maintain a healthy body weight. Scientific reports show men with BMI of 30 or higher have an increased colon cancer risk. (For more on how the body develops high levels of insulin in the blood and insulin resistance, see chapter 13, "Pancreatic Cancer.")

Some evidence suggests why abdominal obesity (as opposed to weight carried on hips and thighs) poses a greater risk for colon cancer. Abdominal fat is linked to especially high levels of insulin as well as insulin-related growth factors that can promote tumor growth. Men tend to carry excess weight around their middles, thus their cancer risk is increased.

As many obese women tend to carry excess weight on their hips, thighs, and buttocks, other mechanisms may be involved regarding their risk for colon cancer. It's possible that in the future, a waist-to-hip ratio (for circumference measurements) will predict women's colon cancer risk. Although few studies have been published with comparisons of these ratios with cancer risk, one such study found an increased colon cancer risk among women with high waist-to-hip ratios—but only among inactive women. This suggests that regular exercise may counter abdominal fat's cancer-promoting effects.[15]

Obesity, Physical Exercise, and Cancer

Observational studies suggest that physical activity can prevent cancer, although there have been no controlled clinical trials on cancer risk and exercise. Sufficient evidence exists, however, to show that avoiding excess weight prevents a variety of cancer diseases, including colon, breast (in postmenopausal women), endometrial, kidney (renal-cell carcinoma), and esophageal (adenocarcinoma) cancers.

The amount of physical activity needed for health benefits adds up to about a half hour daily in total and does not require a trip to the gym. Any lifestyle activities that keep people moving are recommended, and these can include gardening, biking, walking, playing sports, dancing, doing odd jobs or housework, and taking the stairs instead of the elevator. For many people who are overweight, decreasing their calorie consumption while increasing their daily physical activities may be all that is needed to reach a healthy weight. Documented scientific data show that regular physical activity can reduce the risk for several types of cancer.[12]

For people with severe obesity (a BMI greater than 40), it may not be possible to exercise efficiently or to exercise at all. Some studies suggest that bariatric surgical intervention (comprising a variety of procedures) could save these people from several life-threatening diseases such as diabetes, hypertension, and certain types of cancer—but these surgeries also can have serious complications. This kind of medical intervention should be considered only on the recommendation of physicians.[18]

Breast Cancer

Studies have found that exercise can reduce the risk for breast cancer as well as other cancer diseases. Most studies on exercise and breast cancer risk have been conducted with postmenopausal women, so more research is needed on the topic of exercise and breast cancer risk for women in other age groups. One study shows that postmenopausal women who walk 30 minutes daily have a 20 percent lower risk of breast cancer. Women who maintain a healthy weight have even more benefits: a 37 percent decrease in cancer risk. However, the researchers found that women who were seriously obese did not experience exercise's protective effect.

Colon Cancer

Exercise appears to have a powerful effect on colon cancer risk—possibly lowering the risk for this cancer by up to 50 percent, according to observational studies. The exercise need not be particularly vigorous, either. One study demonstrated that three to four hours weekly of brisk walking lowers colon cancer risk. How exercise benefits the colon is not well understood, although various biological mechanisms may be involved, such as energy balance, immune system regulation, insulin level regulation, and encouragement of the steady progression of bodily products through the gut. Although colon cancer rates appear to be reduced by regular exercise, no consistent scientific data yet show a reduction of rectal cancer risk associated with physical activity.

Pancreatic Cancer

Some research indicates that people who are obese have an increased risk for pancreatic cancer. This may be due to the direct relationship between obesity (BMI of 30 plus), abdominal fat deposits, and insulin production. Ample evidence demonstrates that intra-abdominal fat is involved in developing insulin resistance. This insulin resistance and the abnormal glucose metabolism that can accompany obesity without diabetes may also be pancreatic cancer risk factors.

Researchers have found that physical activity may reverse this effect by reducing intra-abdominal fat, thus possibly increasing insulin sensitivity. Physical activity has been found to improve glucose metabolism, boost insulin activity, and lower plasma insulin levels in addition to its effects on body weight. This suggests that obesity and abdominal weight gain may be modifiable risk factors for pancreatic cancer and that these risk factors may be reduced by physical activity. Researchers have also noted less pancreatic cancer incidence among people who exercise compared with people who are mostly sedentary. And so moderate physical activity may have an inverse relationship with pancreatic cancer risk.

CANCER PREVENTION

Biological Mechanisms for Physical Activity

Physical activity helps protect the body from disease mostly by changing metabolic hormone levels and growth factor activity and by decreasing body fat and possibly enhancing the immune system.

Some evidence shows that increasing physical activity lowers the body's levels of insulin, glucose, and triglycerides while bumping up HDL cholesterol (sometimes called good cholesterol) levels. All these beneficial changes may help reduce the cancer risk. Exercise also increases production of a protein known as insulin-like growth factor binding proteins (IGFBPs). As suggested in their name, these IGFBPs bind to insulin-like growth factors (IGFs) circulating freely in the body and render them inactive. As IGFs promote cell or tumor growth, one of exercise's many benefits may be to slow or stop tumor growth.

Lowering one's caloric intake also increases production of IGFBPs, with beneficial results similar to exercise's. Conversely, someone who lives an inactive lifestyle and who eats high-calorie foods will have a higher risk for breast, colorectal, lung, and prostate cancers.[12]

Insulin Activity Moderation

One way physical activity reduces cancer risk is by adjusting insulin activity. A metabolic hormone, insulin plays an important role in preserving energy balance, but problems with this hormone can have a big impact on health. For example, defects in insulin pathways can lead to insulin resistance, a risk factor for type 2 diabetes.

The chain of events that is insulin's cellular activity begins when the hormone binds to insulin receptors on the cell's surface. Inside the cell, insulin receptors are then activated via phosphoylation (a type of chemical modification), which then gathers intermediates, including insulin receptor substrates (IRSs). This series of actions (or insulin signaling) results in an increase in growth factor production and, therefore, cell proliferation. It also results in an increased presence of cytokines, such as proinflammatory cytokines.

This means that obese people who have insulin resistance and associated type 2 diabetes also have increased levels of proinflammatory cytokines. As discussed in the section on obesity and chronic inflammation later in this chapter, activation of the inflammatory pathway may be a factor in the higher incidence of cancer in obese people.

Oxidative Stress Reduction

Oxidative stress is another factor that may trigger inflammation in people with obesity. This occurs after high insulin levels spark an increase in glucose delivery to adipose (fat) tissue. The fat tissue's endothelial cells then may take in rising amounts of this simple sugar. In hyperglycemic conditions (excess blood sugar), the endothelial cells' rise in glucose intake creates an excess production of reactive oxygen species in the cells' mitochondria. As a consequence, the cells experience oxidative damage, and inflammatory signaling is activated. Inflammatory cells (macrophages, for example) may also be drawn to these damaged endothelial cells, worsening the inflammation. Even more inflammation develops because of hyperglycemia, as this state sparks production of reactive oxygen species in fat cells. This in turn leads to a higher production of proinflammatory cytokines.[16]

As exercise lowers the body's insulin levels, it also decreases a number of downstream cancer-promoting effects that may happen when insulin is out of balance.

Lower Levels of Free-Circulating Steroid Hormones

Increasing physical activity may also reduce hormone-related cancer risk by decreasing the amounts of free-circulating steroid hormones (mostly androgen and estrogen) in the body. These types of cancer include endometrial, breast, and prostate cancers. Several researchers have demonstrated that higher levels of circulating estrogens in postmenopausal women, especially if they are obese, are linked to a higher breast cancer risk. This cancer risk may be more elevated if these women have also had more long-term exposure to endogenous estrogen hormones. The long-term estrogen exposure may be caused by an increased number of ovulation cycles due to, for example, early onset of menstruation, giving birth for the first time at a late age, no lactation, or menopause occurring at a late age.

On the other hand, vigorous exercise may offer women protection from hormone-related cancers, as lean women and girls who participate in high-intensity physical activities such as gymnastics or ballet have reduced levels of circulating estrogens. Exercise may also lower estrogen in postmenopausal women by decreasing adrenal androgen conversion to estrogen. But it is not yet known how much exercise is needed or the specific time periods in life for exercise to most help decrease endogenous sex hormone production.

Sex hormone levels pose a risk for not only women but men. Prostate cancer risk may be predicted by endogenous hormone level too, as research has shown that increased plasma testosterone levels are accompanied with an increased prostate cancer risk.

Yet, once again, exercise appears to counter this effect. Scientists have noted that increased physical activity is linked to higher amounts of circulating sex hormone binding globulin in men and women. Sex hormone binding globulin lowers endogenous levels of estrogens and androgens after competitively binding to these sex hormones.

Genetic factors will also influence how well exercise prevents cancer for any particular individual. Factors such as capacity for conditioning, body build, and physical ability may affect people's risk for various cancers on an individual level.[12]

Obesity and Chronic Inflammation

As described above, adipose tissues are active endocrine organs that encourage production of metabolic hormones, such as insulin and leptin, and proinflammatory cytokines, the markers of inflammation. Research using transgenic (genetically altered) mice shows that many genes involved in inflammatory pathways have higher expression levels (of gene transcripts RNA or protein) in obese mice than in normal-weight mice. This suggests that obesity is connected with chronic inflammation.

As scientific evidence shows that leptin, insulin, cytokines, and bioactive lipids all play roles in the body's immune response and energy balance, a link may also exist between energy balance and immune response.[12] These systems use some of the same cellular mechanisms, and the metabolic (energy balance) and immune systems also regulate each other. Thus, there are parallels in these two pathways (particularly in cytokines) so that when there is an infection there is an alteration in cytokine expression. Often, infection and inflammation are accompanied by increased fat metabolism (as a form of metabolic support) to provide the necessary cytokines to fight infection and inflammation.[16]

As noted, several key molecules help oversee metabolic function as well as immune response. The hormone leptin has an essential role in maintaining the body's energy balance, but it also functions in adaptive (learned response) and innate (immediate generalized response) immunity. Studies show that a lack of leptin impedes immune function in mice as well as in people. As metabolism and immunity are linked, lowered leptin levels may explain the immunosuppression associated with starvation in some parts of the world. For example, researchers learned that mice who were starved for two days—and who had become immunosuppressed—experienced an immunosuppression reversal when they were given leptin. Meanwhile, lipids themselves also assist in the regulation of inflammation and metabolism.[12,16,19]

More on the immune system and cancer will be discussed in the next chapter.

Scientific evidence demonstrating that metabolic imbalance leads to immune imbalance is accumulating. The above example of the connection between immunosuppression and starvation shows what happens at one extreme of the metabolic-immune system partnership. At the other end, we find obesity and inflammatory diseases.

While a lack of vital nutrients, or worse, starvation, dampens immune function and makes people more vulnerable to infection, obesity creates a state of abnormal immune activity and inflammation in the body. This raises the risk for a wide variety of inflammatory illnesses such as airway inflammation, fatty liver disease, diabetes, and atherosclerosis.[16]

Physical activity, particularly endurance training over the long term, enhances immune function. This means higher numbers and activity of macrophages (white blood cells that attack pathogens), natural killer cells, and other infection fighters in the immune system's arsenal, all discussed in chapter 19, "Immune System and Cancer Risk."

Calorie Restriction and Cancer

Eating slightly less than what one would naturally consume is an old technique for extending life. Scholarly papers often credit Lucretius (ca. 50 B.C.) with being the first to have suggested that rampant eating leads to premature aging and degenerative diseases.

The old Roman poet was on the right track. Scientific evidence shows that restricting calories (called calorie restriction), or undernutrition without malnutrition, significantly decreases the risk for age-related diseases and may even delay death. Researchers found that yeast, worms, flies, mice, and rats that were put on calorie-restricted diets had considerably longer lives than their control counterparts.

Some researchers demonstrated that rhesus monkeys fed 30 percent less calories for 20 years experienced much slower aging processes as well as less age-related diabetes, heart disease, and cancer than the control group. These calorie-restricted monkeys looked younger, too. Other studies have shown that animals on calorie-restricted diets usually are sleeker, healthier, and more vibrant than animals allowed to feed at will (most of these animals gained weight in midlife).

Calorie restriction continues to intrigue scientists as, so far, it is the most widely investigated and successful experimental strategy for maximizing the longevity of mammals. This approach to eating also seems to be the most effective and far-reaching dietary intervention for cancer prevention seen in experiments.[17] Calorie restriction should not be mistaken for malnutrition or starvation, a common error that may have prevented some useful research findings from being incorporated into population disease prevention strategies long before now.

When correctly designed, a calorie-restricted diet features essential nutrients and vitamins but carefully controlled total energy consumption. Calorie decreases of about 20 to 30 percent (compared to free-feeding tendencies) can still be seen as a normal, healthy level of food consumption. While the people who benefit the most from calorie restriction may be those who have followed this approach throughout their lives (as opposed to beginning as an adult), adopting this eating approach in adulthood may still prevent obesity and a host of diseases, suppress tumor growth, and extend lifespan.

Experiments have shown calorie restriction's longevity effect in people. Researchers learned that reducing caloric intake in Spanish nursing home residents lowered morbidity and mortality. One step or two past calorie restriction is another dietary approach of interest: fasting. This approach delivers even more pronounced physiological changes related to those seen in calorie-restriction diets. It may be that fasting's cleansing and detoxifying effects make it the most beneficial natural healing therapy. Fasting has long been part of many spiritual and religious traditions, including Christianity, Judaism, and Eastern religions. It is a spiritual purification rite that can greatly improve one's physical health, too.[13]

Mechanistic Targets of Calorie Restriction

Experiments focusing on energy balance and genetic susceptibility in mice demonstrated that calorie restriction offered several significant benefits: the diet decreased tumors, increased tumor latency, and reduced serum insulin-like growth factor and leptin levels. In most tissues studied, animals that had a calorie-restricted diet had reduced cell growth. This slower pace of DNA duplication in healthy cells may mean these cells are less vulnerable to carcinogen-induced

DNA damage. The calorie-restricted diet also suppressed the proliferation of mutated cells. Thus many of the antiaging benefits of adopting a calorie-restricted diet may be due to the reduced cell proliferation, which delays the appearance of cells that may produce genes that promote predisposition to age-related diseases, including cancer.[17]

Calorie restriction offers more antiaging and anticancer benefits, including reducing oxidative stress and inflammation. This may be due to calorie restriction's limiting effect on free-circulating insulin-like growth factors, as well as on the production of reactive oxygen species in the body. Reactive oxygen species are a by-product of regular bodily functions such as energy metabolism, antipathogen immune response, cell death regulation, intracellular signaling, and other processes. But the accumulation of these oxidants, particularly as a by-product of metabolism or response to inflammation or environmental stress (tobacco smoke exposure, for example) is associated with cancer development, tumor growth, and other age-related diseases in mice, nonhuman primates, and people.

Thus, limiting food consumption through calorie restriction may help prevent some of the oxidative damage associated with aging—as well as disease.

SUMMARY

The numbers of overweight and obese people in the United States and other developed countries are skyrocketing. Consequently, the incidence rates for many chronic obesity-associated diseases such as diabetes, heart disease, and most cancers are also climbing.

Whereas obesity can promote tumor growth, studies using genetically altered mice indicate that a nutrient-dense, calorie-restricted approach to eating can suppress tumor development and offer many other antiaging benefits. Exercise—even mild activity such as gardening, walking, or housework—also comes out a winner for the multiple ways it prevents disease and promotes health. Physical activity has also been found to enhance immune function, and as immunity is linked to metabolism, both of these key systems benefit from regular activity.

Exercise and dietary adjustments may not be strong enough medicine for some people with severe obesity, however. In some cases, surgical intervention may be needed to reduce body fat and improve health.

Immune System and Cancer Risk

A healthy immune system is essential for a healthy life—and to avoid cancer. Deficient immune systems put people at increased risk for certain types of cancer as well as other diseases. In fact, scientific studies estimate that up to 15 percent of cancer incidence around the world is related to microbial infection. This suggests a firm link between weak immune systems, chronic infection, and cancer. Common examples of this connection between chronic infection and cancer are the human papillomavirus, associated with cervical cancer, and the hepatitis B and C viruses, which are linked with liver cancer.

Some people's immune systems fail to recognize their own tissues, as a result triggering autoimmune diseases. Certain medications that suppress the immune system (such as are used after organ transplantation) are associated with a higher risk for cancer diseases, including leukemia and cervical cancer. Defective immune systems may contribute to a higher cancer risk in several ways. They may allow opportunistic infections to take hold, such as Kaposi sarcoma, a possible consequence of infection with human herpesvirus (HHV8) infections. Or immune systems may respond inappropriately as a secondary response to infections such as *H. pylori* in the stomach, giving rise to a higher risk for gastric cancer. In general, conditions linked to chronic irritation and the ensuing inflammation, such as through long-term exposure to tobacco smoke or workplace irritants such as asbestos, may dampen immune reaction and can make the body more vulnerable to cancer development.

THE FUNCTIONING IMMUNE SYSTEM

All multicellular organisms have an immune system to fight off microbial infections. This includes plants, invertebrates, and vertebrates. The human immune system is a sophisticated and intricate web of cells, tissues, and molecules that work together to neutralize threats to bodily health. It strives to prevent new infections while destroying established ones.

The immune system has two main points of defense: innate immunity and adaptive immunity. Innate, or natural, immunity refers to the protective factors one is born with. In healthy people, innate immunity is always ready to block microbe entry and to launch an attack against microbes that have entered bodily tissues. Adaptive, or acquired, immunity is stimulated by invading microbes, adapts to this new target, and forms a response that becomes learned after a few days.[1]

A key function in a healthy immune system is the ability to recognize the human body's own tissues, to separate self from nonself, so to speak, and eliminate invaders. Appropriate targets include infectious organisms such as bacteria (streptococci, for example), fungi (*Candida,* a cause of yeast infections), and parasites. Because of the variety of infectious agents the body encounters, the immune system must utilize a wide range of defensive mechanisms to destroy invaders. Problems occur, however, when the immune system deploys these destructive powers against the body's own tissues.

In a healthy body, the immune system serenely coexists with other bodily cells. Human nonimmune cells ensure this by producing certain marker proteins on their surfaces that the immune system recognizes and tolerates in a state of "self-tolerance." These markers are unique to each person and are called the major histocompatibility complex (MHC). Nonself substances lack these specific markers; those that provoke immune response are called antigens. These can be whole cells from other organisms, a bacterium, a virus, or possibly an MHC marker protein (or part protein) from a foreign organism.

Antigens, of course, have their own markings, called epitopes. These trigger immune response through the immune system's agents, proteins referred to as antibodies (immunoglobulins). These antibodies recognize antigens by their nonself epitopes and neutralize them. This is why the immune system rejects organ or tissue transplants. MHC molecules are a blueprint for the immune system to recognize and protect the body's own cells, as well as a means of identifying infectious invaders.

INFLAMMATION

The immune system's actions against an antigen flare up in a process known as inflammation, the result of a complex cascade of events that target foreign objects for destruction. In a nutshell, the system works like this: first, circulating blood platelets identify an antigen (it may be a bacterium, virus, irritation, or trauma to the body). The platelets surround the antigen and release platelet-derived growth factor to attract white blood cells and other lymphoid cells. Next, the infection-fighting white blood cells arrive and release cytokines, chemokines, prostaglandins, and leukotrines to begin the repair process and prevent further invasion.

Some of these white blood cells are natural killer cells, special immune cells constantly on the lookout for foreign invaders and infected cells. As their name suggests, these natural killer cells do not need any prior experience with antigens to target them. Natural killer cells are potent foes of viral infections and other antigens—even cancer cells.

Two of the immune system's key weapons are agents that produce antibodies called B lymphocytes and agents that seek out and eliminate pathogen-infected cells called T lymphocytes. As part of the adaptive immune system, these lymphocytes take action several days after the initial infection. They launch a specifically designed attack using information received from antigen-presenting cells, such as dendritic cells (which act as messengers between the innate and adaptive immune systems).

The T lymphocytes coordinate the immune response and destroy viruses or other antigens hiding in infected cells. When antigens are found that match up with antigen-specific antibodies on B lymphocytes, the antigen binds to the antibody receptor and the B lymphocyte engulfs it. The body has a vast number of B cells, each with specific receptor binding sites for its recognition antigen (which fit together like a lock and key), all floating around in the blood until they encounter antigens.

Meanwhile, a helper T lymphocyte assists in attacking the antigen, until it is demolished and consumed by macrophages (large white blood cells that digest foreign invaders or damaged tissues).

DEFECTS IN THE IMMUNE SYSTEM

As the immune system's main purpose is to protect the body against infection, defects in its machinery can mean leaving the body vulnerable to everything from the common cold to potentially fatal diseases such as cancer. A defective immune system gives rise to disorders known as immunodeficiency diseases. These can be caused by mutations in important regulatory genes in immune function. A few examples of these genetic abnormalities are described below.

As discussed earlier in this chapter, the immune system has an essential mechanism to prevent the body's immune defenses from attacking itself. If this mechanism breaks down, the body can develop a variety of autoimmune diseases. Or perhaps the immune system's device for recognizing infections fails. In this case, the body begins to produce T lymphocytic cells and antibodies that attack its own tissues and organs. This can lead to autoimmune diseases as well as other diseases and disorders. For example, T lymphocytic cells directed against cells in the pancreas play a part in diabetes, while an autoantibody (antibody directed against self) called the rheumatoid factor is often found in rheumatoid arthritis sufferers.

GENETIC SUSCEPTIBILITY AND IMMUNITY

The immune system neutralizes most viral infections, yet some infections persist and, worse, cause cancer. Genetic predisposition may be to blame. As viral infections are thought to induce nearly all cases of cervical cancer (as well as other cancers), some researchers speculate that a defective gene could be responsible for some people's inability to clear the infection. However, if this were true, the hypothesis is that cervical cancer patients would likely carry a wide variety of mutations influencing the gene's activity. For example, some people who have difficulty in resolving viral infections have mutations in the *RNASEL* gene that are linked to lower RNASEL activity. These mutations are also associated with several cancers, including breast, cervical, familial prostate, and more aggressive pancreatic cancer.[2]

Studies suggest that altered cytokine (intercellular signaling peptides) levels may at least in part be a heritable risk factor. One possible example of this is Hodgkin lymphoma, the hallmark of which is immune dysfunction. Other research has shown alterations in *Th1* and *Th2* cytokine genes that can change gene behavior, alter the balance of responsiveness between these cytokines, and affect predisposition for infectious disorders, autoimmune diseases, and cancer.

This could have a big impact on health as cytokines are essential to the regulation of key immunity pathways. Th1 (cell-mediated) cells help fight viruses and other pathogens as well as help remove cancerous cells. Th2 (humoral) cells oversee humoral immunity by boosting antibody production against pathogens or free-floating foreign molecules (antigens). In fact, the correct Th1-to-Th2 ratio is vital for maintaining the optimum immune surveillance of the body. A ratio skewed toward Th2 is linked to increased likelihood of allergies, asthma, and autoimmune disease. A balanced ratio of Th1 and Th2 cells is maintained by a specific group of proteins known as cytokines (which are regulated by growth factors).

As immune dysfunction may contribute to the development of lymphoma, an imbalance in the workings of Th1 and Th2 cytokines (called the fundamental messengers of adaptive immunity) may be a risk factor for non-Hodgkin lymphoma. Genetic variance in cytokines known to be involved in the immune system could explain health-related differences in different ethnic groups.[3]

THE IMMUNE SYSTEM AND CANCER

After normal cells become cancerous, some of the protein markers, or antigens, on the cells' surface may be altered. (In healthy cells these are recognized as self, except in autoimmune disease.) This is often seen in cells from tumors that arise from cancer-inducing viral infections. These viruses may manufacture antigens that the body will recognize as foreign; the immune system's job, then, is to locate these cancerous cells and obliterate them before they become dangerous.

The fact that the body's immune system can target a tumor suggests that tumors must manufacture antigens that the immune system knows are foreign (or nonself). This particular defense mechanism is called immune surveillance, and evidence shows that this activity is essential for preventing tumor development. One theory suggests immune cells are continuously monitoring the body, watching for and eliminating cells that have become cancerous.

Some tumors do not express (manifest) foreign cell surface antigens; instead they overproduce antigens, or their process for regulating expression of these antigens is dysfunctional and attracts attention from the immune system.

So one may well wonder why cancer is so common if the body's immune system is able to identify and destroy tumors. But cancer is a formidable opponent. To fight cancer, the immune system must find and destroy all tumor cells and so must patrol vigilantly. Tumors are opportunistic and develop when immune surveillance breaks down. It may be that, once caught, these tumors have had enough of a start to overpower the immune system's defenses.

Several other factors may prevent the immune system from efficiently eliminating all tumor cells. For example, cancer cells may very closely resemble healthy cells and may not be noticed by the immune patrol. Or the immune system may have one or more defects, as described above, that make some people more susceptible to certain kinds of cancer.

A more insidious reason is that some tumors develop qualities that help them avoid immune detection. They may stop expressing antigens that attract immune attack. These tumors are known as antigen-loss variants, and if the lost antigen is not needed to continue the cancerous properties of the tumor, these variant tumor cells grow and multiply. Other tumors stop producing the major histocompatibility complex (MHC) molecules, so they no longer present antigens for the immune system to locate.

Tumors may also avoid immune system detection by losing their antigen expression, by turning off molecules needed for antigen processing or expression of MHC molecules, or by releasing cytokines that have a dampening effect on immune response.[4]

MECHANISMS THAT LINK INFLAMMATION AND CANCER

As noted earlier in the chapter, the immune system uses inflammation to spark a healing response to infection or tissue injury. The inflammatory process is useful; it can repair damaged tissues and even encourage tissue regeneration. Yet research shows that the chronic inflammation that develops because of chronic irritation may contribute to cancer initiation and growth. Therefore, cancer is like a wound-repairing process that has gone wrong.

Normally, inflammatory chemical manufacturing stops when the tissue is healed. But if cancer forms, these chemicals continue to be produced without end. This leads to chronic inflammation through the functions of inflammatory mediators such as tumor necrosis factor alpha (TNF-α) and interleukin (IL-6 and IL-17). Excessive production of these proinflammatory chemicals can impede immune response and therefore speed tumor growth and development.

The tumor's microenvironment features a fine balance between antitumor immunity activity and the tumor's own proinflammatory activity. Whether the tumor or the immune system gains an edge depends on the different mediators unleashed by body's inflammatory cells, the tumor cancer cells, and other varieties of tumor-associated host cells.

If the immune system's antitumor activity falls short of the tumor's immunosuppressive activity, tumor cells are free to grow and multiply. If the body's antitumor immunity is stronger than the tumor's immunosuppressive actions, then the tumor cells are destroyed. Research indicates, however, that the net outcome of a chronic inflammation in the microenvironment speeds tumor growth, progression, and expansion into surrounding tissues; formation of new blood vessels to feed tumor growth; and metastasis.[5]

Usually the presence of leukocytes and other signs of inflammation seen at tumor sites indicate a pathogenic infection. Yet other signs of inflammatory response have been found in breast and prostate cancer tumors where infection is not considered part of the cancer risk. Many of these types of tumors contain proinflammatory cytokines and macrophages, in addition to a gene expression profile (gene activity patterns) with an inflammatory signature. (As cancer cells may show heightened gene activity in relation to the immune inflammation response, this is called an inflammatory signature.)

While macrophages are part of the immune system's arsenal, tumors are sneaky and can mimic normal cells to evade detection and destruction. These so-called tumor-associated macrophages have been reprogrammed, or altered, by the cancer cells so that they have little cytotoxicity for the tumor cells.

A higher risk for prostate cancer is linked to genetic defects in the macrophage signaling pathway, whereas the presence of proinflammatory cytokines from chronic inflammation is linked to the greater potential for mammary (breast) epithelial cells to invade other areas of the body. However, studies on transgenic mice that lack a proinflammatory enzyme show they have delayed onset of breast cancer. These data support the hypothesis that inflammation contributes to the initiation and possibly the progression of cancer.[6]

The success of nonsteroidal anti-inflammatory drugs in preventing spontaneous tumor formation (in people with familial adenomatous polyposis) also supports the growing evidence that cancer and inflammation are related.[7]

DIET, IMMUNE SYSTEM, AND CANCER

As discussed earlier in this chapter, a person may become predisposed to cancer after any environmental exposure that provokes chronic inflammation, which weakens immune response. Furthermore, some highly active components of the immune system such as lymphocytes continuously produce reactive oxygen species (ROS) as part of their normal function. These ROS molecules can harm cellular membranes, cellular proteins, and nucleic acids as well as promote chronic inflammation. Therefore, any means that helps prevent chronic inflammation in the body may also help prevent cancer.

Nutritious foods are full of bioactive components that can perk up the immune system by reducing inflammation and, as a result, reduce the cancer risk. As discussed more thoroughly in chapter 17, "Nutrition and Cancer," fruit and vegetables are full of beneficial phytochemicals and vitamins. The antioxidants vitamins C and E and carotenoids, flavonoids, and minerals such as zinc and selenium can bind to ROS, inhibiting oxidative damage.

The omega-3 polyunsaturated fatty acids DHA and EPA are also sources of helpful antioxidants. Carbohydrates that are sources of beta-glucans (polysaccharides), found in the cellulose of plants and some kinds of fungi and cereal grain bran, can activate the immune system and may have antitumor activity. Shiitake mushrooms, oats, and barley are a few examples. Other evidence is adding up to support the theory that probiotics and prebiotics affect immune response and may offer cancer prevention.

More knowledge is needed about bioactive food components, especially of their potential to prevent cancer. It may be that specific amounts of certain nutrients would be more beneficial than others or that some people have different nutritional needs for cancer prevention.[8]

Phytochemicals are some of the most powerful immunomodulators (substances that affect the immune system). Particular fruit and vegetables may contain polyphenols, curcumin, or isothiocyanates that may have cancer-fighting properties. (The role of fruit and vegetables in cancer prevention is discussed more thoroughly in chapter 17, "Nutrition and Cancer.")

Scientists have identified several cancer-busting chemicals found in broccoli and cabbage. An example is 3,3'-diindolylmethane (DIM)—a chemical produced from the compound indole-3-carbinol after cruciferous vegetables such as cabbage, broccoli, and kale are eaten. Laboratory studies with animals have demonstrated that DIM can halt the development of particular cancer cells. DIM may also perk up the human immune system.

Other research has indicated that DIM stops breast cancer cells from dividing and limits testosterone (the male hormone needed for prostate cancer cell growth). Studies have also shown that DIM boosts blood cytokine (immune cell regulators) levels, which may have a beneficial effect on the immune system.[9]

EXERCISE AND IMMUNITY

Studies have shown that natural immunity is improved during moderate exercise, but after long-term, rigorous exercise, immunity may be compromised. This is because long periods of exhaustive activity appear to suppress the cells involved in eradicating infected cells and tumor-target cells. This suggests that moderate exercise protects against cancer but intense exercise does not. At present, the data that support this hypothesis is very limited.[10]

Exercise exerts considerable physiological changes in the immune system. The evidence shows that exercise alters the body's hormone levels, inciting blood concentrations of stress hormones to climb during vigorous, intense muscular activity. These hormones include the flight-or-fight hormones epinephrine and, to some extent, norepinephrine, as well as the stress hormone cortisol (during a long workout). The presence of these hormones adds to the acute effects on lymphocyte subpopulations as well as on natural killer cell activities. These increase in the blood after exercise, too.[14] Thus, acute, intense muscular exercise boosts testosterone and estrogen concentrations,[15] whereas prolonged physical exertion (marathon running, for example) decreases testosterone levels.[16]

But during moderate exercise, levels of the sex hormones testosterone and estrogen may be reduced, possibly boosting immunity. This may be because these hormones help control lymphocyte (including natural killer cells) activity. So after not-too-intense exercise, the immune cells are strengthened, coming back stronger and more aggressive.

Exercise also enhances immune response and raises production of cytokines to attend to an injury or infection. These cytokines help direct incoming lymphocytes and other healing cells to clean out antigens and begin tissue healing.

Exercise's effect on hormones and the immune system is complex, but overall, exercise is an important modulator of immune function.

STRESS, IMMUNE SYSTEM, AND CANCER

A person's stress level and emotional well-being have significant effects on ability to fight diseases such as cancer. Several studies indicate the negative effect of stress on the human (and animal) immune response. Energetic, happy, and relaxed people tend to be less likely to catch colds—and are less prone to complain about the colds and flu that they do catch than angry, depressed, or nervous people. This research suggests that a positive outlook may boost the immune system's ability to fend off infection.[11]

It is not yet known exactly how positive emotions or a stressfree lifestyle enhance individual immune systems—or how negative feelings depress the natural defenses. But scientific evidence suggests that positive emotions may influence health through physiological arousal.

For example, researchers have demonstrated that cold symptoms arise from the release of chemicals such as cytokines, histamines, and bradykins as a result of an infection. To some degree, hormones such as oxytocin control these chemicals. It may be that positive feelings are linked to the release of these chemical-controlling hormones, while negative feelings and stress do not prompt such a release.

Happy and otherwise pleasant feelings also spark immunoglobulin A secretion and a reduction in salivary cortisol, although the lower cortisol secretion does not necessarily imply that a person is feeling less stressed. (One small pilot study examined stress reduction and lower cortisol and did not find a significant association.[17]) While the mechanisms underlying how positive emotions from the brain interact with the immune system are not understood, it may be that different emotions lead to different types of physiological stimulation in the brain. Multiple hormonal pathways may exist between the brain and the immune system and may become activated in response to this stimulation or physical infection or injury.

Recent research supports the theory that people with negative mind-sets have a poorer immune response and may be more at risk for illness than people with more sunny mind-sets.[12] In one study scientists noted that medical students under stress during examinations took longer to manufacture proinflammatory interleukins (immune system infection fighters) and were slower to heal wounds than other medical students who were not stressed.[13]

These results show that psychological stress may have an impact on the gene expression patterns of key proinflammatory genes needed by the immune system to fight infection. Other research shows that people with chronic stress have lower levels of natural killer cells than people who have less stress. As natural killer cells are some of the immune system's most powerful infection fighters, lower levels mean lower defenses. This suggests that if stress lowers the body's defenses, the body also loses its ability to conquer cancer cells.

SUMMARY

The body needs a healthy immune system to fight deadly illnesses such as cancer. Studies show that when cancerous cells evade the immune system, usually they do so by taking over the immune system's defensive inflammatory response mechanism for fighting infection. In a bit of biological irony, cancer uses the human body's defenses to promote disease development.

While not all the mechanisms are understood, studies suggest that a complex combination of factors influence the immune system's efficacy at fighting cancer and other diseases. These factors include diet, exercise, brain stimulation, and emotions that may affect the immune system via the brain.

Natural approaches may be effective at reducing cancer risk in this respect. By eliminating or reducing exposure to proinflammatory toxins in the environment, adopting an anticancer diet, seeking emotional balance, and staying relaxed and calm through exercise, you can reduce chronic inflammation and therefore the risk for disease.

Chapter 20

Controversies Concerning Cancer Screening's Benefits and Disadvantages

Time and again, the scientific evidence shows that a commitment to a healthy lifestyle may prevent cancer. A few key examples include eating nutritious food, exercising regularly, and avoiding tobacco smoke.

Some people, however, may be more prone than others to developing cancer. This may be because of inherited genetic mutations or exposures to toxic environmental factors such as radiation or other unidentified risk factors, particularly if the exposure happens in childhood or infancy. So even if a person takes precautions and makes lifestyle changes to avoid cancer, he or she may already be predisposed to develop the disease later in life.

In the quest to reduce cancer deaths, scientists have developed screening methods to detect early-stage cancers to improve the chance of a cure. But over the past few years, a number of controversies have erupted over whether the benefits of screening outweigh all the possible associated drawbacks, some of which are considerable. This topic is discussed further in this chapter. First, let's have a look at screening.

SCREENING AND EARLY DETECTION

People who undergo screening are usually without symptoms. They are given diagnostic tests or procedures with the hope that early detection of a cancer will mean they are more likely to respond to treatment and be cured. Screening tests are used not to diagnose cancer but find red flags such as lumps or abnormal cells. If any are found, then more tests usually follow to look for cancer. An example of this is the mammogram that finds a lump in breast tissue: more tests are needed to determine if the lump is benign or cancerous.

Yet in spite of many advances, the science of cancer prevention and detection remain among medicine's most controversial topics. A major challenge is that it can be difficult to determine if a particular cancer will advance rapidly, progress more slowly, or possibly, not develop at all. In many cases, people who have an indolent cancer or a benign disease will die from other causes before they die from cancer, so detection and treatment are unnecessary and offer no benefit whatsoever. Worse, the treatment could itself cause unnecessary stress, harm, even disfigurement. Slow cancers, by their dawdling nature, frequently have a longer presymptomatic period, increasing the likelihood of discovery and improving the chances of treatment. These cancers may be well worth catching. With particularly aggressive cancers, the disease can move so quickly that early detection and treatment cannot help.

Another factor influencing outcomes is that the attitude people have about cancer may help decide whether they live or die (and how quickly) from the disease.

The goal, then, in cancer screening is to determine who would benefit the most from early detection. The good news is that scientists are getting closer to identifying specific gene expression signatures that may help predict if cancers will be aggressive or not.

SCREENING CONTROVERSY

Currently, health care organizations offer varying cancer screening test guidelines. The recommendations may differ by cancer type, the type of screening tests, or how often the tests should be done. This issue became more confusing in 2009 after the release of revised and highly controversial cancer screening recommendations by the U.S. Preventive Services Task Force (USPSTF), an independent panel of government-financed experts that reviews clinical preventive health care services. As an example, this group recommended against routine mammograms for most women in their 40s and suggested that women of average risk consider getting mammograms every other year from age 50 instead of annually. The USPSTF also recommended against teaching breast self-examination, mostly because of false positives leading to more doctor visits, biopsies, and anxiety.[90]

These recommendations, and others, were hotly debated in the media by medical experts and health organizations. The American Cancer Society maintains that women of average risk should continue to get annual mammograms from age 40. Its chief executive officer, John Seffrin, released a letter to the press (October 23, 2009) confirming the society's position on screening and adding, "Yet we have long acknowledged that cancer screening isn't perfect. Sometimes cancers get overlooked. Sometimes cancers get misdiagnosed. Sometimes aggressive cancers can appear even after a clear screening test. It is important to acknowledge these limitations, understand them, discuss them with your doctor, and decide what is right for you."

SCREENING GOALS

In general, screening recommendations have several goals. First, the disease must be considered a public health threat. Second, the screening test should identify disease at an early stage, when people undergoing the test are yet without symptoms and while a cure may still be possible. In other words, the test should ultimately lead to a lower mortality rate. This also means that people who are diagnosed after a positive screening test must have access to effective treatment. Together, effective screening tests and treatments can decrease a disease's impact on public health.

Third, tests should be safe, cost efficient, and able to identify the disease's absence as well as its presence in people. And last, the benefits of screening must be greater than the risks. For example, the rate of false positives and false negatives must be weighed against the possible advantages of the test. Incorrect findings can be costly in many ways. False positives can lead to unneeded surgeries, unneeded treatments, stress, and public health costs. False negatives can mean disease goes undiscovered, possibly progressing past the point when treatment could be beneficial.

As the key point of cancer screening is to reduce illness and death, screening must improve health outcomes, otherwise the purpose for screening is lost. It may seem counterintuitive, but early detection alone is not a good reason for a screening program. Screening programs benefit the public only if early detection (and the consequent diagnosis) can ultimately improve public health; this requires that adequate treatment be available for found diseases and that false test results have a low incidence.[1]

These concepts help illustrate the context for the present controversies surrounding screening recommendations. This chapter describes current views and debates on screening for breast, cervix, colorectal, lung, and prostate cancers, diseases that account for more than half of all cancer deaths in the United States. (Discussion on the contemporary controversies around nutrition and food supplements follows in chapter 21 as well as a look at the questions regarding certain environmental exposures in chapter 22.)

SCREENING FOR PROSTATE CANCER

As the second-leading cause of cancer-related death in men (after lung cancer), prostate cancer has a deadly impact on the U.S. public.[2] It is the most common nonskin cancer found in men and its incidence has been increasing, although some of the rise in prostate cancer rates may be because of testing based on prostate specific antigen (PSA) levels. More on that topic further on.

Prostate cancer can be treated successfully if discovered early. It is slow growing, but this disease can create a painful death if left untreated. So as prostate cancer is clearly a major health problem for men, the advantages of screening leading to early detection and successful treatment are obvious. But a number of points are relevant here. The screening techniques for prostate cancers are not as sensitive or specific as could be desired. For example, some people may have normal PSA levels but harbor prostate cancer, while others with a higher PSA may not have prostate cancer.

Prostate cancer also tends to be an age-dependent disease. Researchers studying organ donor samples from men who died from a variety of causes (including stroke, car accidents, and gunshot wounds) discovered that prostate cancer incidence increases after age 40 and rises dramatically after age 50. They noted an approximately 33 percent chance for prostate cancer in men ages 60 to 69, and a 46 percent chance for prostate cancer in men ages 70 to 81.[3]

Other studies have found that at least 95 percent of new diagnoses and 97 percent of prostate cancer deaths happen to men older than 60 (the median age is between 75 and 79 for incidence and mortality). Thus this disease usually strikes people with a relatively limited life expectancy.

Moreover, compelling evidence shows that treatment for prostate cancer found through screening inflicts moderate to substantial harm. This can include impotence, incontinence, and possibly death. The potential for negative consequences is particularly troubling as many of these men with prostate cancer detected through screening may never have had any cancer-related symptoms develop during their lives.

Prostate Cancer Screening Tests

Three screening tests are currently used: digital rectal examination, circulating PSA, and transrectal ultrasonography. Most studies on these tests' effectiveness have been conducted with men who already had cancer symptoms, although clinical studies are ongoing. In general, it's been found that these tests are good for detecting late-stage disease but not sensitive enough for detecting most early-stage cancers.

Digital Rectal Examination

Digital rectal examinations (DREs) are used to check the prostate (located beside the rectum and within the body) for the lumps, enlargement, or hardness that may indicate disease. The data show that DREs have a limited sensitivity for finding organ-confined and possibly curable cancer. One reason for this is that the examiners can feel only part of the prostate and so can miss abnormalities. This screening technique detects about 30 to 40 percent of identified prostate cancers. Because of this, some researchers have questioned the value of DREs as a routine test done by general practitioners.

Transrectal Ultrasonography

Transrectal ultrasonography is a costly method that uses inaudible sound waves emitted by a probe inserted into the rectum to create an image of the prostate and surrounding tissues. This technique rarely finds prostate cancer that a DRE and PSA screening cannot find. Consequently, this method is often used to guide biopsy but not for routine testing.

Prostate Specific Antigen

A PSA test measures PSA levels in the blood, which may be higher in men who have prostate cancer. PSA is a key serum marker for prostate cancer and has helped detect more of the clinically and pathologically confined cancers. But this marker has also contributed to a great many false positive results. As described below, recent studies in Europe show a statistically significant lowering of mortality rates as a consequence of PSA-based screening—although this was accompanied by an increased risk of overdiagnosis (diagnosing diseases that may never manifest symptoms or otherwise harm the patient).

It's important to note that the circulating PSA test measures the risk for prostate disease, not prostate cancer itself. A variety of diseases of the prostate affect PSA levels and, therefore, screening results. These diseases include prostatitis (inflammation of the prostate gland), benign prostatic hyperplasia (enlarged prostate), and infection, as well as prostate cancer. Prostatic manipulation (the act of massaging the prostate) can also increase PSA levels.

Also, while a PSA test may offer more sensitivity than DREs, these tests are still not sensitive enough to use alone. In 1994 the U.S. Food and Drug Administration (FDA) approved circulating PSA tests to be used together with DREs to screen for prostate cancer. But while blood PSA levels above four nanograms per milliliter (ng/mL) are considered abnormal, and marked for further testing (such as a biopsy), about 25 percent of men with localized prostate cancer have PSA levels that are below that threshold and considered normal.

Up to 15 percent of men age 50 and older have blood serum PSA levels greater than 4 ng/mL, with cancers found in 25 to 30 percent of them. As mentioned above, high PSA concentrations are also found in men with enlarged, inflamed, or infected prostate glands—common conditions in older men. In fact, about 25 percent of men with benign prostatic hyperplasia have PSA levels ranging between 4 and 10 ng/mL, some with serum concentration levels as high as 15 ng/mL. So while a lower cutoff level for PSA concentration (less than 4 ng/ml) would improve the test's sensitivity (more men with prostate cancer would be detected), it would also reduce specificity (more men with PSA-raising conditions other than prostate cancer would be targeted).

Consequently, the PSA-based screening technique leads to many false positive and false negative results, and it is not a reliable method for the early detection of prostate cancer. The data show this testing method has a sensitivity of 90 percent but a specificity of only 10 to 31 percent.[4]

More research and study is needed to enhance this method's sensitivity and specificity, as well as to determine the positive predictive value of a variety of cut-off PSA concentration levels. PSA screening needs to become more sophisticated so that benign prostate disease is not mistaken for prostate cancer and so that it is possible to determine clinically significant prostate cancer.[5]

At present, several factors weigh against screening. These include illness or injury as a result of testing (particularly biopsies); the anxiety and stress caused by false positive results; the illness, injury, and death caused by unnecessary treatment of those diagnosed with incurable prostate cancer; and the discovery of clinically insignificant disease with the accompanying upset and stress. It's because of issues like these that scientists conduct randomized controlled trials to learn whether prostate cancer screening actually reduces mortality.

In Europe the results from such randomized clinical trials indicate that PSA-based screening does offer benefits but perhaps to only a small percentage of men (a similar randomized trial in the United States is currently underway). Initiated in the early 1990s, the European randomized study to evaluate prostate cancer screening with PSA testing found a statistically significant drop in the rate of death from prostate cancer as a result of PSA-based methods. The study randomly assigned more than 162,000 men ages 55 to 69 to a group that received PSA screening every four years or to a control group that did not get screened. The researchers noted that the screened group had 20 percent fewer deaths compared to the control group. Nevertheless, the absolute risk difference was 0.71 deaths per 1,000 men—or less than 1 man per 1,000 men. This means that 1,410 men would have to be screened and 48 more cases of prostate cancer would have to be treated (possibly needlessly) to stop 1 man from dying from prostate cancer.[6]

Of course, to that one man in more than a thousand and his friends and family, cancer screening is hugely beneficial. The study clearly shows potential benefits but at an enormous cost in money and in the numbers of men who must be treated to find the overall health benefit. For that reason, the study results suggest that men should carefully consider whether to have a PSA-based screening test. Men in high-risk groups may wish to minimize their chances of dying from prostate cancer and will choose to have a PSA test. Otherwise, men may not see any advantage in undergoing PSA testing, considering the benefit-to-risk ratio is so small.

As the recommended guidelines for prostate cancer screening differ between organizations, the decision to screen or not tends to fall on which guidelines individual urologists follow. Here are a few samples: the American Cancer Society and the American Urological Association recommend that physicians offer annual

DREs and PSA screening to men age 50 and older who have at least a 10-year life expectancy and to younger men at higher risk for prostate cancer. The Canadian Task Force on Preventive Health Care and the USPSTF do not recommend DREs or PSA screening for the general population. The American College of Physicians recommends doctors discuss the potential benefits and known harms of screening, diagnosis, and treatment with the patient to come to an individualized decision.

Some doctors suggest that men who have an especially increased risk—such as those with multiple first-degree relatives diagnosed at an early age—should start getting tested at age 40. On the other hand, the USPSTF does not recommend the regular use of PSA testing in men older than 75. The reason is that the potential harm done as a result of PSA testing on men in this senior group outweighs the benefits. This evidence also demonstrates that the incremental benefits for men age 75 and older are small to nonexistent when it comes to treating cases of prostate cancer found through screening.

Not enough evidence currently exists to show if health outcomes are better for men age 75 or younger who were treated for prostate cancer following screening, compared to men who were treated for cancer following clinical detection.[7]

SCREENING FOR BREAST CANCER

Breast cancer, the most common nonskin cancer for women, is the second-most-frequent cause of cancer death in women. It also tends to strike women fairly early in their lives and so causes more lost years of potential life than all the other cancers. Thus breast cancer meets the criteria for screening. Mammography-based screening is now the most common test for this disease; other methods include clinical breast examination, breast self-examination, and magnetic resonance imaging (MRI).

Mammography

Mammography is a type of x-ray test used to find small lesions or abnormalities in breast tissue to identify women who may be at risk for breast cancer. Although this method of screening is very commonly used, concerns over its effectiveness have sparked heated controversy among medial professionals and health organizations. Study results have been varied: some studies found that mammography screening benefited health outcomes, while other studies found no benefits.

This shows the importance of conducting randomized controlled trials to find out if mammography-based screening for breast cancer can lower death rates. Scientists in the United States and other Western countries have performed several such randomized clinical trials with more than 600,000 women ages 40 to 74 years. These trials did not show evidence for any real advantages to mammography for women ages 40 to 49 years old. However, for women in the 50 to 69 age group, mammography screening was shown to reduce death from breast cancer by about 30 percent. The studies have little data for women ages 70 to 74, but the available evidence shows nearly no difference in the outcomes of women who had mammography screening compared to those who did not.

Some of the effects of the debate on mammography and these studies can be seen in the differing guidelines, as mentioned above regarding the screening controversies and the USPSTF. Although organizations and health professionals continue to have opposing views, the studies suggest that regular screening mammography in the 50-to-74 age group does reduce breast cancer–related deaths. In women ages 40 to 49, the evidence in support of screening is not as clear. Yet without a doubt, breast cancer is a significant cause of illness and death among women in this age group.[8]

That said, using mammography as a screening tool also involves some risk: radiation exposure (although small), false negatives, false positives, emotional upset and financial costs, the possibly uncomfortable examination, and the possibility of overdiagnosing ductal carcinoma in situ (the most common type of noninvasive breast cancer) and risking overtreatment. The goal is to detect the small fraction of ductal carcinomas that are aggressive, but this diagnosis can also pick up otherwise-indolent ductal carcinomas that would not have created illness. It is often not possible to pinpoint which women do not need medical intervention.

Rates for false positive mammogram results are as high as 6.5 percent. False positives mean unnecessary follow-up visits for mammography and biopsies as well as anxiety and stress.

As with prostate cancer screening, to improve the specificity of breast cancer screening some studies found that using two methods together might improve results. In this case, clinical breast examination used along with mammography may be an improvement on using mammography alone—although whether the costs of combined screening are outweighed by its benefits is still controversial.

Yet other studies have found that women who have had a decade of screening have a one in three chance of false positive results from breast cancer screening. This includes a 24 percent chance of a false positive mammogram and a 13 percent chance of a false positive clinical breast examination. Naturally, this tends to upset people and boost the number of patient-initiated doctor visits. Because of all these uncertainties, women should talk with their doctors about the risks and benefits of mammography screening.[8,9]

Clinical Breast Examination

Clinical breast examination (CBE) is a doctor's physical examination of the breast. Before the recent controversy, this breast cancer screening method was recommended for women ages 20 to 39 to have at least once every three years, then every year after age 40, and even more often for women at high risk. As with mammography, this type of breast cancer screening also has shown false positives. So far studies suggest it is no more sensitive than mammography. It's possible that having a clinical breast examination would be more beneficial during the years women do not have a mammogram.

As breast cancer is not limited to women, anyone of either gender who finds breast lumps, nipple discharge, asymmetric thickening, or changes in breast skin should see a doctor.

Monthly Breast Self-Examination

Self-examinations are a breast cancer screening technique used by women or men to check their breasts for lumps or other irregularities. The American Cancer Society and other advocates recommend this method as a cheap test that is ultimately worthwhile. Yet the results of three randomized trials done in countries without mammography screening indicate that this technique has no statistically significant effect on breast cancer detection, nor was it found to reduce death from breast cancer. As noted above, the USPTF recommends against teaching women to perform this test.

SCREENING FOR LUNG CANCER

Lung cancer continues to be the number-one killer of men and women. In 2010 an estimated 222,520 Americans were diagnosed with this illness and another 157,300 died from the disease, according to figures from the National Cancer Institute.[113]

Lung cancer is hard to treat once the disease has spread to other areas in the body. Thus the overall five-year-survival rate for all lung cancers is only about 15 percent. This changes dramatically for lung cancers caught in their earliest stages, for which the five-year-survival rate is up to 70 percent. As more than 90 million people in the United States smoke or have smoked, providing an effective screening test along with effective treatment would have a huge impact on public health. Yet as we have seen with other screening methods, the present lung cancer screening strategy has generated plenty of controversy.

Chest X-ray and Sputum Cytology

Chest x-ray and sputum cytology are typically used together in efforts to screen for lung cancer. Randomized screening trials designed to evaluate these screening methods did not find that either test was successful in reducing death due to lung cancer.[10]

Computed Tomography or Helical CT Scan

Computed tomography (CT) scans are an imaging technology that can find lung cancer with more sensitivity and at an earlier stage than chest x-ray and sputum cytology. The CT scan gets its greater accuracy from taking several x-ray images and merging them into a computer image. This technology can detect tumor lesions smaller than one centimeter. X-rays can be used to find lesions down to only one or two centimeters in size.

Observational studies have found that people with lung cancer detected by CT scans have increased survival rates. Yet some reports show a high proportion of false positives as this screening method also finds noncancerous abnormalities. Still, ongoing studies have not yet established if finding these smaller tumors leads to fewer deaths from lung cancer. One ongoing randomized clinical trial, the National Lung Screening Trial (NLST) sponsored by the National Cancer Institute, compares the results of CT scans and chest x-rays to establish if either screening method can lower lung cancer death rates. Other smaller randomized clinical trials are underway in Europe and will be compared to NLST results.[1]

While the use of helical CT scans (faster, more sensitive, three-dimensional versions of the standard, two-dimensional CT scans) for lung cancer screening sounds promising, the possible negative consequences from overdiagnosis cannot be left unnoted. These include mental and emotional upset due to false positive results as well as illness and possible death due to chemotherapy and other medical interventions. And all these terrible effects might be suffered for tumors found through CT scan screening that may never have progressed into life-threatening, symptomatic illnesses.

Another problem is that noncancerous abnormalities are not so unusual. Recent research shows that 20 to 60 percent of smokers' and former smokers' CT scans will locate irregularities. The majority of these are often areas of inflammation, scars caused by smoking, or other conditions that are not cancerous.

Genomic Data

Genomic data, used along with current lung cancer screening and diagnostic tests, is a new and promising approach to lung cancer prediction.[11] A genomic data test looks for changes in 80 genes found in patients' airways, with the goal of finding out which smokers may develop cancer.

Usually, after an imaging test shows an abnormal mass in a smoker's lungs, the next step will be a bronchoscopy. In a bronchoscopy, a thin tube with a camera is sent down into the person's lungs to check for irregularities and take biopsy samples. However, bronchoscopy detects stage I lung cancer in only 15 to 20 percent of cases. This means that to find out if the detected lesions are cancerous, doctors often must follow up with more costly and invasive tests such as exploratory surgery. This is often where doctors may look at the available evidence and make the decision to either recommend more invasive tests or monitor the patient for the time being. As of yet, no biological markers or established diagnostic tests can determine which smokers have lung cancer.

Enter genomic testing. Smokers' airway cells are examined for abnormal patterns of gene activity that are linked to lung cancer. The idea behind the test is that cigarette smoke carcinogens will likely affect gene behavior throughout the respiratory tract, not just in the abnormal mass detected through screening. Alterations in gene activity then can have diagnostic uses.

Researchers hope to identify gene activity patterns that will help them separate smokers with lung cancer from those without the disease. Results reported in 2007 demonstrated that the combination of genomic test with bronchoscopy make for better predictions of lung cancer than either test on its own.

These combined tests may increase detection of early-stage cancers that are often missed by bronchoscopy but are more likely to respond to treatment. Still, the 80-gene signature test is experimental and needs to be validated in scientific studies. Currently, a trial is in the works to evaluate this genomic test in 300 people in Europe and the United States. If proved to be effective, genomic testing should speed up the process for more invasive testing and suitable treatment for smokers with lung cancer. It should mean fewer invasive diagnostic tests for people who do not have lung cancer.

SCREENING FOR CERVICAL CANCER

The Pap Smear

The Pap test, or smear, named after the scientist who developed it, George Papanicolaou, is used to detect cervical cancer and may be the most successful cancer screening program. In this test, a doctor collects cells from the cervix during a routine examination. These cells are later examined for abnormalities that may indicate precancerous or cancerous changes.

While apparently no randomized controlled trials have been conducted to demonstrate its effectiveness, a review of historical data from British Columbia, Canada,[39] shows 80 percent fewer deaths from cervical cancer between 1955 and 1988, credited to the province's organized public Pap screening programs. In other countries with national screening programs such as the United States, Pap tests have cut cervical cancer death rates by more than half since the 1960s, when this test became commonly used.[1] Unfortunately, many women who do not have access to screening continue to die from cervical cancer.

On the negative side, the Pap test is not an especially precise tool and may miss underlying precancerous conditions, so most women must continue to have regular tests until late in life. When part of routine gynecological examinations, the Pap test will eventually reveal abnormalities or precancerous lesions before serious disease sets in. So as frequent testing is needed to protect women from cervical cancer, the resultant costs for medical programs are high. This has been a source of some debate. However, scientists are seeking new methods, to help reduce the expense of this valuable screening tool.

VACCINES THAT CAN PREVENT CANCER

The Human Papillomavirus Vaccine

As discussed in chapter 4, "Cervical Cancer," the development of the human papillomavirus (HPV) vaccines opens up the possibility of preventing cervical cancer around the world. It is a great step forward for women's health. But the issue is certainly not free of controversy.

The vaccines are designed to protect women from HPV types 16 and 18, the carcinogenic viruses that induce 70 percent of cervical cancers, and HPV types 6 and 11, the infections that cause 90 percent of genital warts. However, as these vaccines are preventive measures, not cures, they cannot treat an already present HPV infection. This means that to be effective these vaccines must be given to women before they are infected with an HPV virus. As many women become infected with some type of HPV on their first sexual experience, scientists recommend that very young women or girls be vaccinated to achieve the maximum benefit. This, of course, creates several dilemmas for parents, such as whether to have their young daughters vaccinated and how to explain the vaccine's purpose to their daughters if they decide to proceed.

Because of all the issues HPV vaccines raise, parents need to learn about HPV, cervical cancer, and HPV vaccines. An understanding of all the facts is necessary to make an informed choice regarding immunization. Older women, meanwhile, may already have come in contact with HPV when they are vaccinated so would very likely need to continue with Pap testing.[12]

HPV Vaccine and Men

Epidemiological evidence shows that women are at a higher risk for cervical cancer when they have sexual partners who have had multiple sexual partners. A woman's risk for cervical cancer also increases with the number of extramarital affairs her husband pursues. While the main goal of the HPV vaccines is to prevent cervical cancer, men would benefit from HPV vaccination as well. Men can experience significant consequences from an HPV infection, as the virus is linked to a higher risk for head and neck cancer, among other diseases. Therefore, men should also share some of the responsibility of research and the possible advantages of vaccination. If men were to be vaccinated for HPV, this would greatly boost the public health benefit of the vaccine.

SCREENING FOR COLORECTAL CANCER

Colorectal cancer is clearly a significant disease: it is the second-leading cause of death by cancer for Americans, according to the American Cancer Society.[114] At age 50, a person has a 5 percent lifetime risk for colorectal cancer and a 2.5 percent chance of dying from the disease. It's interesting that three-quarters of all people newly diagnosed with this disease have no known risk factors (other than age).

Randomized controlled trials have shown that screening for this cancer through fecal occult blood testing (FOBT), described below, results in a statistically significant drop in colorectal cancer deaths. Yet while this screening test is effective, it is underused in the United States. That's despite health insurance plans usually paying for this type of screening.[1]

Several tests are used to detect colorectal cancer in its early stages, including FOBT, digital rectal examination, colonoscopy, barium enema (as an alternative to colonoscopy), and sigmoidoscopy. These tests tend to be given to people older than age 50, although people in high-risk groups may begin screening earlier. Colorectal cancer risk factors include a family history of colorectal cancer, polyps, inflammatory bowel disease, and in women, a family or personal history of breast, endometrial, or ovarian cancer.

Fecal Occult Blood Test

FOBT is a screening test that detects blood in stool samples. Blood may be a sign of colorectal cancer, although it may also be caused by hemorrhoids, colon polyps, peptic ulcers, or anal fissures. This is why the FOBT is a screening tool, not a diagnostic test.

Sigmoidoscopy

Sigmoidoscopy is a test usually given following a positive FOBT. It involves the insertion into the large intestine of a flexible tube with a fiber-optic camera to check for abnormal growths, such as polyps, that could become cancer. This type of screening is controversial as case-control studies support its use but no randomized controlled trials have been conducted yet.

Colonoscopy

Colonoscopy often follows a positive result from other screening methods, as when tumors such as tubular adenomas are found because these benign tumors can become cancerous. Two recent studies involving people without symptoms suggest that this form of test is more sensitive to key signs than sigmoidoscopic testing. The trials found that for participants with advanced proximal neoplasms (abnormal tissue growth or tumors) found during colonoscopy at least half had no distal abnormalities. These would likely not have been caught by sigmoidoscopic testing. The results suggest that colonoscopy would find many more precancerous cases or cases of colorectal cancer in its early stages than sigmoidoscopic testing on its own.

Yet other studies indicate that colonoscopy would not benefit people with tumors smaller than five millimeters that would not develop into polyps.[13] Hence, the goal is to match up people with whichever test would benefit them the most—even both tests, if needed.

Another factor in this mix is the cost of screening. Some reports put the screening cost of saving one life at $300,000. But as no studies have yet proved that screening tests result in fewer deaths, the question about whether colorectal cancer screening saves lives is still unanswered.

Genetic Screening for Cancer

Genetic screening is commonly used to detect chromosomal abnormalities. For example, pregnant women who may be at risk for carrying a baby with genetic irregularities often undergo a type of prenatal genetic testing called amniocentesis. In this test, a sample of amniotic fluid is withdrawn to check for fetal chromosomal abnormalities. Likewise, people of African ancestry may have blood samples genetically tested to check for an autosomal recessive disorder (disease caused by mutations in two copies of same gene) called sickle-cell anemia. Others, particularly those of Caucasian European ancestry, may require genetic testing for the autosomal recessive disorder cystic fibrosis.

Thanks to advances in human genetic research, cytogenetic (cellular aspects of heredity) screening can be used to check for chromosomal abnormalities. These include mutated DNA and chromosomal translocation (chromosomes abnormally rearranged), which are linked to a higher risk for cancers, including breast, colorectal, and leukemia.

The Human Genome Project, an international effort to uncover the sequence of the chemical base pairs that form DNA, has had (and will continue to have) a profound impact on our knowledge of the genetics underlying disease. It comes down to four nucleotides—adenine, guanine, cytosine, and thymine—that are arranged in different combinations to make about 100,000 genes. Close to 30,000 are understood as encoding for structural and functional proteins. When any of these are misread, the action of a protein can be either suppressed or increased or can possibly lead to the creation of a faulty protein and, consequently, diseases such as cancer.

Examples include several mutated genes known to increase susceptibility for cancer, such as the *BRCA*1 and *BRCA*2 genes that raise the risk for breast cancer. Or the gene mutations involved in Lynch syndrome (also known as hereditary nonpolyposis colorectal cancer, or HNPCC) that greatly increase the risk for colon cancer as well as other cancer diseases.[14] Both of these examples and others are discussed in more detail in earlier chapters, which also include plenty of discussion on how mutations and chromosomal abnormalities have been shown to raise the risk for a variety of cancers.

New Tests for Cancer

New technology and knowledge promise new approaches, and it appears that soon scientists will be able to use a panel of biomarkers to detect disease in its earliest stages. Cancer shows distinct gene expression patterns in tumors when compared to noncancerous tissues, hence these patterns may serve as red flags to signal a cancer's presence. These red flags could be genetic mutations, changes in gene expression, or gene promoter activity. Using DNA microarray technology, it's now possible to measure the expression of thousands of gene transcripts in a single experiment.

Recently, scientists have been investigating the potential of blood tests for cancer. Cancer cells, as well as DNA and RNA shed from these cells, have often been found in the blood of cancer patients (an indication that the cancer has spread or is about to)—something rarely found in healthy people. Using the new technology, scientists may be able to use these biomarkers to find cancer in blood serum, urine, saliva, or other bodily fluids.

For example, microarray-based analysis is being investigated to see if it's possible to test urine for bladder cancer.[91] Another study looked at the potential for blood tests to detect circulating cancer cells showing several gene expression patterns in the blood of breast cancer patients.[92] Yet other researchers have examined the disease-detecting and monitoring potential of altered DNA methylation patterns found in cancer-related genes in the saliva of patients with head and neck cancers.[93]

But while biomarker-based detection tools have been developed for many types of cancers, very few have been explored for large commercial use. This is because these new biomarkers require careful randomized testing and long-term studies to evaluate their effectiveness as sensitive and specific cancer detection tools—and whether the benefits of their use outweigh potential costs.

However, the goal of an effective cancer blood test may be a step closer due to a recent announcement from scientists from Veridex and Johnson & Johnson Ortho Biotech Oncology. They have developed a microchip-based screening tool to detect circulating cancer cells in the blood that may have potential for mass production and detection of cancer.[94,95] A readily available blood test for cancer would revolutionize cancer diagnosis and, potentially, treatment, depending on the ultimate sensitivities of such noninvasive tests.

The completion of the Human Genome Project has had wide-reaching effects and promises a new age of genetic information and technological advances that may ultimately lead to disease prevention and better human health. But as with many advances in science, the new genetic knowledge and possibilities also bring forth fresh ethical, legal, and social issues. For example, genetic information could be used by insurance companies to turn down applicants or deny access to health care or treatments. Or employers could use genetic information to avoid hiring people (or to release others from employment) with certain inherited traits. Because of the potentially far-reaching risks attached to this new knowledge, the U.S. Congress and other government bodies around the world have taken action to prevent the abuse or misuse of genetic information.

Groundbreaking Genetic Nondiscrimination Law

In the United States in 2008, the Genetic Information Nondiscrimination Act was enacted to prohibit employers and health insurance providers from using genetic information to make a variety of decisions related to firing or hiring and health coverage eligibility. This law is meant to protect genetic privacy as well as allow people to take full advantage of the latest genetic developments in both health care delivery and research.[17] In short, this law protects information about genetic tests, family members' genetic tests, and the manifestation of a disease or disorder in family members. It also protects information about a person's or family member's involvement in genetic testing, counseling, or educational research.

To fully benefit from the Human Genome Project, scientists need to know how best to use the new genomic information in making decisions about genetic testing. The genetic tests and other technologies must be used appropriately and must be reliable, sensitive, and specific—and above all, worthwhile.

At present, the American Society of Clinical Oncology recommends genetic testing in these circumstances: the patient has a personal or familial history that suggests a genetic cancer susceptibility condition, the test can be interpreted sufficiently, and the results will help in diagnosis or affect the medical approach used for the patient or the patient's family.

The family of a person considering genetic testing is also important, as the genetic information involves them, too. During the genetic counseling process for cancer, the entire family's medical history is recorded. This will show whether the patient and family members will have an increased risk for particular cancers. But shared genes do not necessarily mean shared genetic information. This can create dilemmas for patients and doctors alike.

Genetic testing, however, can offer advantages whether the results are negative or positive. A negative result means the relief of no more tests or surgery, while a positive test may lead to catching the disease at an early state when successful treatment or a cure is possible. Depending on the outcome of the screening, a physician or a medical geneticist would be in the best position to discuss options for managing or preventing cancer risks.

Scientists, meanwhile, are studying different genes that may be linked to familial predisposition to other types of cancer. The goal is to broaden the capability of genetic screening and prevent disease.

GENETIC SCREENING FOR COLORECTAL CANCER

Genetic causes for colorectal cancers are rare, accounting for less than 10 percent of people with colorectal cancer. Two of these uncommon conditions known to predispose people to this cancer are familial adenomatous polyposis and Lynch syndrome.

Familial Adenomatous Polyposis

Familial adenomatous polyposis (FAP) generates numerous polyps (or adenomas) in the colon that can become cancerous. By the time carriers of the mutation are between ages 15 and 20, hundreds of these polyps will have formed in their colons. While one polyp may have a fairly low risk of becoming cancerous, people with this condition have so many polyps that colon cancer is almost guaranteed by middle age.

Almost all cases of FAP are due to a genetic mutation in the *APC* tumor suppressor gene. This gene encodes for a protein thought to be critical in cell adhesion, signal transduction, and transcriptional activation. As many as 300 different mutations of this gene in FAP cases have been noted. People suspected to be carriers of this mutated gene can undergo DNA-based mutational studies for the *APC* gene.

Hereditary Nonpolyposis Colorectal Cancer

Hereditary nonpolyposis colorectal cancer, or Lynch syndrome, is another familial genetic condition that greatly raises the risk for colorectal cancer. Caused by mutations in genes responsible for DNA mismatch repair, people with Lynch syndrome have an up to 80 percent lifetime risk for colorectal cancer (slightly higher in men than women), although the mean age of diagnosis is 44. The mutated gene's inheritors are also at an increased risk for stomach, pancreatic, brain, hematopoietic, endometrial, and ovarian cancers.

A minimum of four genes used for DNA mismatch repair (*hMSH2*, *hMSH6*, *hMLH*1, and *PMS*2) have been found to cause predisposition to Lynch syndrome. Other DNA abnormalities called microsatellite instability (MSI) may also be connected. (It is possible that DNA repair pathway defects produce MSI in DNA.) In family members with Lynch syndrome, 90 percent of colon tumors have MSI. In people with sporadic colorectal cancers, only 15 percent have MSI in their tumors.

Interestingly, researchers have recently discovered that MSI, as a marker for the mismatch repair pathway of colorectal cancer, is linked to better survival rates, stage for stage, in those people with sporadic colorectal cancer who show MSI in their tumors.

Genetic Testing for Colorectal Cancer Predisposition

People who have a strong family history of Lynch syndrome–related cancers or FAP can be tested to see if they carry the DNA mutations. This may involve a DNA-based mutational analysis from colon biopsy tissue samples or from blood samples from the patient and a family member for evidence of mutations in particular genetic markers.

The advantages to genetic testing for carriers include learning about their risk for cancer as well as the need for routine screening to catch the disease in its earliest stages. Early detection of polyps reduces the risk of death from colorectal cancer, thus this type of screening could be very valuable. For example, Lynch syndrome mutation carriers are typically recommended to have annual or biannual colonoscopies from age 20 or 25 or starting 10 years earlier than the earliest age that colorectal cancer has appeared in a family member.

People who have had positive test results for the mutated gene in Lynch syndrome typically undergo regular colonoscopy examinations, and more than half of them describe the procedure as unpleasant or even painful. A controversial strategy for the carriers of this mutated gene to consider is prophylactic colectomy (surgical removal of the colon), which has its own difficulties and challenges.

Of course, people may benefit greatly from genetic testing if they learn they are not carrying the mutation and are spared from further invasive, expensive, and often uncomfortable screening examinations.[15]

While genetic testing for Lynch syndrome and FAP offers multiple advantages, several issues can complicate the decision to test. First, while colorectal cancer screening has been shown to be effective, the effectiveness of screening and other risk-reduction strategies is not yet known for other Lynch syndrome–related cancers. Second, people considering genetic testing to establish their cancer risk also need to consider the effect on their families: whether family members will want to know the results and the potential for upset and conflict in the process.

Furthermore, people may be concerned that learning they have the genetic mutation may affect their (and their children's and other family members') access to life insurance or subject them to some other discrimination. Governments that are enacting laws regarding genetic information (as noted about the U.S. Congress, above) are still in the process of anticipating and addressing the problems and challenges that may yet arise. Any gaps in this protection could become a problem.

Breast Cancer and Genetic Screening

Predisposition to breast cancer is another rare inheritance, accounting for 5 to 10 percent of the risk for breast cancer. Many of these familial breast cancer cases involve the genes known as *BRCA*1 and *BRCA*2. Studies involving women with an Ashkenazi (eastern European) Jewish background show they have a much higher risk than the general population for this gene mutation. The research has shown that the mutations are passed down through the generations, increasing the risk for cancer in female and male family members. Some researchers estimate that 23 out of 1,000 people of Ashkenazi Jewish descent have *BRCA*1 and *BRCA*2 gene mutations, about five times the rate of the general population.[16] These genetic mutations also increase the risk for other cancers, including endometrial, ovarian, prostate, pancreas, and stomach.

Yet not everyone with these mutations will get breast cancer. This suggests that other factors play a role in breast cancer development. Other unidentified mutations may be connected to familial predisposition to breast cancer.

Genetic Testing for Breast Cancer

When a family has a history of breast cancer or ovarian cancer, it is usually most efficient to test for genetic mutations first a family member with developed cancer. If the *BRCA*1 or *BRCA*2 mutation is found, then other relations can be tested to see if they are also carriers. It's important to note that a positive test result for these gene alterations only shows that a person is at a higher risk for developing cancer. Tests cannot show if a person will get cancer or how well screening or preventive medical procedures will work. As mentioned earlier, not everyone who carries one of these mutated genes will develop cancer.

Genetic screening for those at risk for breast cancer uses DNA-based assays to detect mutations on the *BRCA*1 or *BRCA*2 genes. When faced with a positive result, people can then discuss their individual options with their doctors or geneticists.

SUMMARY

Today, advances in scientific and medical technology can help detect cancers at an early stage when a cure may still be possible, although the efficiency and sensitivity of these tests need improvement. The Human Genome Project's completion promises much in the area of cancer screening through genetic testing, but here again, plenty of work in this field remains to be done as the tests are generally only useful for predicting disease risks and cannot diagnose illness. The genetic tests now available can indicate susceptibility to breast, colon, endometrial, ovarian, pancreatic, and melanoma cancers and can often be performed in clinics or laboratories. As science progresses in human genetic research, it's likely that more cancer prediction tests will be developed and will cost less.

Many questions, however, still need to be addressed about the risk-to-benefit ratio of genetic testing and how it affects research on ethical, legal, and social levels. Once resolved, the benefits of genetic testing and study should be clear—as well as the possibility of eradicating cancer.

Chapter 21

Controversies Surrounding Dietary Supplements and Foods for Cancer Prevention

One strategy to prevent many human cancers is to eliminate or reduce our exposure to environmental carcinogens. Yet complete avoidance of all carcinogenic factors is probably unrealistic. The human body is constantly under siege from a wide assortment of DNA-damaging factors, even from within. Normal metabolic processes can generate potentially damaging free radicals, while inflammation creates oxidative stress inside the body. These factors may spark the formation of cancer or promote the disease's growth.

To the rescue: fruit and vegetables. Evidence from population studies shows that people who eat plenty of antioxidant-rich fruit, vegetables, and grains have lower rates of cancer diseases. The research suggests these edibles can dampen and even reverse cancer development.[18] At present, at least five servings of fruit and vegetables daily are recommended to help prevent cancer, according to the National Cancer Institute and the U.S. Department of Agriculture.[96]

But what if one doesn't eat many fruits or vegetables? Although abundant research and studies confirm the anticancer effects of a diet high in fruit and vegetables, scientists have different opinions on the value of taking vitamin supplements to make up for a lack of plant-based nutrients in daily consumption. Some studies report cancer-preventive benefits from supplementation. Other studies show no benefits and even indicate potential harm—including a raised risk for cancer—from taking high doses of nutritional supplements.

This chapter focuses on the controversies surrounding vitamins in supplemental form versus vitamins found in food and takes a look at consumables with phytonutrients (plant compounds thought to promote health) reputed to help prevent cancer such as green tea and soy. This chapter also examines how dietary fiber may help people avoid disease.

VITAMINS AND CANCER PREVENTION

Vitamin C

Found in fruit and vegetables, vitamin C is one of the most potent antioxidants. Early epidemiological evidence shows that a high intake of vitamin C–rich food leads to a reduced risk for some cancers. Scientists examined 46 epidemiological studies on vitamin C's preventive effect on a variety of cancers; 33 of them identified a strong connection between vitamin C intake and lower cancer rates.[97]

Other research has shown the vitamin's antioxidant power *in vivo*. In 1997 expert panels from the World Cancer Research Fund and the American Institute for Cancer Research suggested that vitamin C can lower the risk for cancer of the esophagus, cervix, lung, pancreas, mouth, pharynx, and stomach. This determination came from an examination of early epidemiological evidence that high consumption of fruit and vegetables rich in vitamin C is associated with a reduced risk for some cancers.[40,115]

Most of this evidence is based on limited observational and interventional evidence, but all in all it suggests that vitamin C intake can lower the risk for cancer.

Vitamin C Supplementation

Randomized controlled trials that featured vitamin C supplementation did not find any decrease in the risk for cancer.[19] Other research suggests that even a low intake of vitamin C (200 milligrams per day) supplements may cause cytotoxic activity in the cell when certain metal ions are present. This may explain why vitamin C supplementation has not been found to be an effective cancer chemoprevention agent.[20]

In fact, a few case reports indicate that large doses of dietary vitamin C supplementation may cause kidney stones, excess iron absorption, birth defects, and even cancer. Because of the present controversies about the benefits and harmful health effects from vitamin C dietary supplements, people should be cautious in the frequency and amount of vitamin C taken. Currently, the U.S. Department of Agriculture and the National Cancer Institute recommend a daily consumption of 200 to 280 milligrams of vitamin C.[107]

How Vitamin C May Prevent Cancer

Vitamin C from food is thought to protect people from diseases such as cancer by scavenging reactive oxygen species (ROS) from cells and by stopping carcinogenic nitrosamines from forming. Hence, the chemopreventive properties of vitamin C are in its mopping up of DNA-damaging ROS and halting cancer initiation or development in the process.

ROS are natural byproducts of normal metabolic function and inflammation caused by oxidative stress. Vitamin C can help prevent harm by stimulating immune function and stopping the metabolic activation of carcinogens. One study demonstrated that vitamin C intake has an inverse relationship with the risk for stomach cancer. Studies involving people at high risk for stomach cancer indicate a protective effect from ascorbic acid, the reduced form of vitamin C.[108]

H. pylori infection is a key risk factor for stomach cancer, and as discussed in chapter 7, "Gastric Cancer," chronic *H. pylori* infection creates the chronic inflammation that may lead to stomach cancer. Vitamin C may mop up the ROS produced by chronic inflammation, thereby reducing the risk for gastric cancer.[21]

While some advocates promote the chemoprevention properties of vitamin C because of its ability to scavenge ROS, this vitamin also has the potential for pro-oxidant activity.[22] This is because antioxidants that are reducing agents can also act as pro-oxidants. Vitamin C has antioxidant properties when it is reducing oxidized substances such as hydrogen peroxide. But this vitamin can also reduce metal ions that then generate free radicals (reducing metal ions is a pro-oxidant property, although it appears that vitamin C behaves predominantly as an antioxidant in the body).[41,42] As an example, vitamin C has been demonstrated to induce the decomposition of lipid hydroperoxides to endogenous genotoxins (agents produced within the body that damage DNA, leading to mutations or cancer) in the absence of transition metal ions. This could lessen the value of vitamin C as a chemoprevention agent.[20]

Vitamin D: Mixed Results

Acquired through sunshine, some foods, or dietary supplementation, vitamin D is important for healthy bones. It may also lower the risk for cancer, according to epidemiological evidence based on randomized controlled trials. In particular, a high intake of vitamin D is linked to colorectal cancer prevention.

Yet in 2006 a randomized, double-blind, placebo-controlled trial of 36,000 postmenopausal women given vitamin D supplementation (400 international units, or IU, per day) with calcium for seven years found no effect on colorectal cancer rates.[23] It may be that, because of the long latency period involved in the formation of colorectal cancer, the clinical study period was too short to show results.

However, the *American Journal of Clinical Nutrition* published a similar trial with dramatically different results. This was a four-year, population-based, double-blind, randomized, placebo-controlled effort involving apparently healthy postmenopausal Caucasian women. The women took a calcium supplement, calcium with vitamin D supplement, or a placebo only. A key difference between this trial and the aforementioned study is the higher amount of vitamin taken, in this case 1,100 IU daily. Women who were given calcium also took higher doses of the mineral than women in the other study. While the researchers aimed to assess bone fracture risk they also studied the data to determine cancer rates. The results showed that boosting calcium and vitamin D intake (even through supplementation) greatly lowers the risk for all cancers in postmenopausal women.[24]

While these results sparked a lot of excitement and interest in scientific circles, the vitamin dose was significantly higher than the current health recommendations. Unfortunately, the study does not include the vitamin D levels, either before or during the study, of the participants who got cancer as opposed to those who did not. More studies are needed to settle this issue.

Yet other studies have examined whether vitamin D has any effect on disease aggressiveness. The researchers of one case-control screening trial (for a variety of cancers) also included an investigation of vitamin D and the risk for prostate cancer.[25] Their results did not show any support for vitamin D lowering the risk for prostate cancer. Instead, some data suggested a higher risk for more aggressive cancer.

One may well wonder after all these inconsistencies if vitamin D offers any real disease-prevention benefits. After all, vitamin D deficiency is frequently seen in people with dark skin pigmentation, in the elderly, and in populations located in higher latitudes. Often no health problems due to lack of the vitamin are apparent in these groups.

Still, plenty of scientific literature supports higher levels of vitamin D being associated with lower overall cancer mortality. While there is convincing data for this association with colon cancer, it is not so clear for breast cancer and other cancers. And so the scientific debate continues regarding appropriate amounts of vitamin D for health. This is because a variety of factors need to be considered, such as a person's vitamin D level, membership in an at-risk group, and the time of year.[43]

Recently, a double-blind, placebo-controlled trial found that vitamin D paired with calcium lowered cancer rates by more than 75 percent.[26] This suggests a strong need for more scientific proof to establish the potential role of vitamin D and good health.

Sunshine, Vitamin D, and Cancer

An odd conundrum presents itself regarding vitamin D and skin cancer. Sunshine is the main source of vitamin D for many people around the world. At the same time, solar radiation is the main cause of skin cancers.

Sunshine contains ultraviolet (UV) radiation in three wavelengths: UVA, UVB, and UVC. More than 95 percent of the sun's UV radiation that lights up the earth's surface is UVA (longer wavelength radiation). The majority of UVC is soaked up by the ozone layer as well as oxygen in the atmosphere and has only a minimal effect on people. Up to 10 percent of the radiation that reaches the planet—and human skin—is UVB. This wavelength has an impact on nucleic acids, proteins, and lipids and can produce DNA mutations that lead to skin cancer.

The UVB wavelength spectrum tans and burns human skin; yet the peak wavelength for DNA damage is nearly the same as what is needed for vitamin D synthesis via the skin. Because of this, it is not possible to have vitamin D synthesis without exposure to the same UVB spectrum that can cause harm.

Excessive sun exposure has a strong association with skin cancer (see chapter 15, "Skin Cancer"), while overwhelming evidence implicates UVB in inducing premalignant skin lesions, in addition to melanoma and nonmelanoma skin cancers.[27]

Vitamin D Supplementation Quandary

Due to the skin cancer risk from excess solar radiation, direct sun exposure should be limited to no more than 15 minutes a day. This may not be enough exposure to synthesize adequate amounts vitamin D, however, so dietary vitamin D supplements may be important for good health.

This is controversial, of course, as vitamin D supplements may not have the same effects in the body as sun-derived vitamin D. Some studies indicate that sun exposure causes the skin to make other photoproducts that may be significant in sun-driven vitamin D synthesis. Fortunately, one can also increase vitamin D intake through food. Good sources include oily fish (wild salmon, for example), eggs, and fortified milk. At present, the Office of Dietary Supplements at the National Institutes of Health (NIH) recommends 600 IU of vitamin D per day for adults aged 19 to 70. The NIH advises 800 IU per day of vitamin D for people older than age 71.[109]

Beta-Carotene

Evidence from animal experiments suggests that beta-carotene (ß-carotene) intake may have anticancer effects, thanks to carotenoid pigments (known for their red-orange tint) that can scavenge highly reactive oxygen species (ROS) and other free radicals. This neutralizes the harmful effects of ROS.

The research history of beta-carotene and cancer illustrates the complexity of showing a causal relationship between nutritional factors and the prevention of disease. Evidence from experiments with animals indicated that beta-carotene intake could have anticancer effects. In vitro and in vivo studies showed that carotenoid pigments were able to scavenge highly reactive species such as oxygen and other free radicals—thereby offering preventive benefits. In the early 1980s, substantial epidemiological evidence already indicated associations between high fruit and vegetable consumption, high estimated beta-carotene intake in the diet, and high blood concentrations of beta-carotene and lower incidences of cancers, particularly lung cancer. Several clinical trials were initiated, particularly the Alpha-Tocopherol and Beta-Carotene (ATBC) Cancer Prevention Study begun in Finland in 1985. Yet the results showed no significant benefits with respect to the prevention of lung cancer, essentially ruling out a primary preventive effect on lung cancer.

Trials published a decade later did not find anticancer effects for supplemental beta-carotene—at least at the doses and duration of vitamin supplementation tested. This is contrary to the findings of observational epidemiological studies. It also suggests that the use of beta-carotene supplementation (in pharmacological doses) will probably not help prevent lung cancer.[28]

Clinical Trials and Vitamin Supplements

All in all, clinical trials investigating the possible benefits of vitamin supplements have not found anticancer effects or reduced cancer risk.

In 2008 the National Cancer Institute reported that selenium and vitamin E did not produce a reduced prostate cancer risk.[98] Launched seven years earlier, this trial involved African American men age 50 or older and Caucasian men age 55 or older (African American men are more at risk for prostate cancer). The participants were randomized to one of four groups, each participant receiving two pills: selenium and placebo, vitamin E and placebo, vitamin E and selenium, or two placebo pills.

A number of earlier laboratory and animal model studies had indicated that vitamin E and selenium had anticancer properties. But the primary spark for this trial was the findings from two cancer prevention trials that indicated that each supplement on its own may reduce the risk for prostate cancer. Thus the National Cancer Institute study was designed to address whether supplements alone or together could affect prostate cancer risk. More than 35,000 men participated. However, an independent review concluded that the effort will not be able to reduce prostate cancer risk by 25 percent (the primary endpoint), and so the men have been asked to stop taking their study pills. They are also asked to continue with the study for another three years in case a longer-term benefit to the supplements regarding prostate cancer risk becomes apparent.

This review also showed an increased prostate cancer risk linked to the supplementation of vitamin E, as well as higher rates of adult-onset diabetes risk following supplementation with selenium, although neither risk was significant statistically.

More rigorous human studies are needed to evaluate the risks of taking high-dose vitamin supplements and to provide proof to the public of any health benefits while justifying nutritional recommendations of supplements. That said, several prospective observational studies show the health benefits of a diet featuring plenty of antioxidant-rich fruit and vegetables. This underscores the general recommendations and old wisdom of eating a variety of nutritious foods.

SOY PRODUCTS AND ISOFLAVONES

Soybeans are one of the most well-researched and richest sources of the phytonutrients known as isoflavones. These isoflavones, including genistein, daidzein, and glycitein, are responsible for most of the humble bean's health benefits. Research suggests isoflavones are powerful antioxidants that may protect against cell damage by mopping up DNA-damaging free radicals. Isoflavones have a chemical structure similar to estrogen and can bind to estrogen receptors; therefore, these antioxidants are known as phytoestrogens.

Soy is a multipurpose food: it can be consumed as edamame (fresh beans in the pod), tofu, soy milk, and miso paste, among other forms. It contains protein and amino acids and has antioxidant properties. And so today soy is a mainstream staple in many countries around the world, showing up on shelves in big-box grocery stores and as milk alternatives in popular coffeehouses. But controversy is brewing along with the soy lattes: soy contains phytoestrogens, so is this food healthy or risky for breast cancer patients and survivors? Does soy protect against cancer or hasten its growth?

ISOFLAVONES AND CANCER:
THE PHYTOESTROGEN CONTROVERSY

Some evidence suggests that as isoflavones may produce estrogen-like effects, they could function as natural alternatives to hormone replacement therapy for menopausal women. However, serum isoflavone concentrations after a high-soy meal can reach low micromolar levels (which are relatively high levels because normal basal serum isoflavone levels are nanomolar, or one-thousandth the concentration of micromolar), thus soy boosts isoflavone levels a thousandfold.

Consequently these estrogen-like effects have also caused some worry that isoflavones may stimulate growth in some kinds of tumors. Results from some rodent model studies seem to support this concern, although these studies tend to use doses of isoflavones that would equal five times the amount found in traditional, soy-rich Asian diets. Also, most of the rodents in this type of research were directly injected with purified isoflavones, giving rise to significantly greater levels of unconjugated isoflavones than what would have been reached through feeding alone. Another issue is that in spite of three decades of research and study, no one has determined the isoflavone dose needed for estrogen-like effects in women. So while these phytoestrogens perform as estrogens in rodent studies, it's not known how much would be needed to show effects in humans.[29]

To sum up, the relationship between soy foods and breast cancer remains controversial because of concerns based mostly on test-tube and animal studies. As mentioned above regarding isoflavones and phytoestrogens, one concern is that isoflavones may promote growth of existing estrogen-sensitive breast tumors.

But soy isoflavones may also behave like weak estrogens and block estrogen receptors. This is how the chemopreventive drug tamoxifen works to prevent a recurrence of estrogen-sensitive breast cancer. Considering the high rate of breast cancer in the United States (about one in seven women will develop the disease) soy could be considered a low-cost, easily adoptable lifestyle change that could reduce the illness and death rates from this disease.

Hence, some researchers believe there is a link between soy consumption and lower breast cancer risk, although this has not yet been proven. Although several studies report that soy intake is associated with a modest reduction in breast cancer risk, inconsistencies across studies limit the ability to interpret these findings.

This conundrum may have a considerable impact on public health because of the increasing popularity of soy foods and the commercial availability of isoflavone supplements.

Little clinical evidence shows a connection between isoflavones and breast cancer risk in healthy women—or a worsened condition in breast cancer patients. Furthermore, the research is limited, but no evidence thus far shows that isoflavones have an effect on breast tissue density or breast cell proliferation in postmenopausal women, regardless of their breast cancer history.

Epidemiological evidence generally agrees with the clinical data, showing no increased risk with isoflavones. Moreover, the clinical and epidemiological evidence appear to show a low overall breast cancer risk linked to pharmacological estrogen exposure in postmenopausal women.

More research is needed to put these concerns to rest, but the current evidence suggests that isoflavone exposure matching typical Asian soy consumption likely does not have a harmful effect on breast tissue. In fact, fewer women suffer from breast cancer in Asian countries (such as Japan) than in Western countries.[29]

Regarding soy's potential as a cancer-fighting food, the National Cancer Institute sponsored a workshop in 1990 that found that soybeans contain components thought to have anticancer properties.[99]

Since then, many scientists have studied soy's reputed capabilities to lower the risk for cancer, especially breast cancer. This disease became a prime interest in this research for a number of reasons. First, Asian women who traditionally eat soy-rich diets have low breast cancer rates—could soy be the reason? Second, other studies suggest the isoflavones found in soy have antiestrogen and cancer-fighting potential. Third, early epidemiological data show an inverse relationship with soy consumption and breast cancer risk. And, lastly, rodent studies demonstrate a protective effect from soy consumption against carcinogen-induced mammary cancer.

The American Cancer Society weighed in on this issue in 2006, concluding that patients with breast cancer could safely eat up to three servings of soy foods daily. But the organization advised against the consumption of isoflavone powders, supplements, or other concentrated sources. Still other experts have voiced their concerns over the use of any isoflavone-containing products for breast cancer survivors or, in some cases, women at high risk for cancer.[44,45]

Meanwhile, a statistically significant inverse relationship was found between plasma genistein (a soy isoflavone) and breast cancer rates in a 10-year Japanese case-control study published in 2008.[30] In other words, the women with the most consistently high levels of soy isoflavone had the lowest rates of breast cancer. It could be that long-term consumption of soy foods offers the most chemopreventive benefits.

Naturally, because of all the conflicting information and advice, many women are confused about whether soy is good for them. Health professionals can help by ensuring they are up to date on the evidence relating to soy and breast cancer so they can better advise their patients. One should note that the U.S. Food and Drug Administration clarified some of the confusion by ruling that 25 grams of soy protein a day is considered beneficial. The FDA adds that consumers must read labels carefully to check for the amounts of soy proteins in food products.[29]

DIETARY FIBER

Dietary fiber is widely thought to lower the risk for colorectal cancer. Recently, a National Academy of Sciences report defined *dietary fiber* to be indigestible carbohydrates and lignin (a complex chemical compound found in plants) that are intrinsic and intact in plants.[100] Nearly all of the fiber a person consumes reaches his or her colon. Dietary fiber may protect this organ in several ways, such as by diluting fecal carcinogens and procarcinogens (as fiber is bulky), speeding up the passage of feces through the bowel, producing the short chain fatty acids that promote anticarcinogenic action, and binding to carcinogenic bile acids.

Yet numerous epidemiological studies examining fiber and cancer risk have had inconsistent results.

On the benefit side of the equation, case-control and ecological correlation studies have found that a high consumption of dietary fiber leads to a low risk of colorectal cancer. For example, statistically significant reductions in colorectal cancer risk were found to be linked to dietary fiber in two recent scientific efforts, the European Prospective Investigation into Cancer and Nutrition study and the Prostate, Lung, Colorectal, and Ovarian Cancer Screening Trials.[101,102]

But most prospective cohort studies have not discovered any link between dietary fiber consumption and colorectal cancer risk. The benefits of dietary fiber supplementation are also unproven: randomized clinical trials of fiber supplements have not shown any connection to reductions in the recurrence of colorectal adenomas (benign tumors that may become cancerous).[31] Still, other studies suggest that eating high-fiber cereals or whole grain foods might lead to some reduction in colorectal cancer risk.

Fermentable Types of Fiber and Cancer Risk

Debate is ongoing in the scientific literature as to whether the fermentation of dietary fiber in the bowel helps prevent or promote colon cancer. Research has shown that poorly fermented fibers are better in vivo dilutors (they create more bulky stools in rodent experiments) as they consequently lower the concentration of carcinogens, procarcinogens, and tumor promoters in feces and cause it to pass more quickly through the bowel. This means harmful substances have less access to the mucous membrane of the colon.

Within the colon, colonic microflora and the physiochemical qualities of the consumed fiber determine its fate. Highly fermentable fiber sources include oat bran, guar, and pectin, while cellulose and wheat bran are less fermentable. The hemicelluloses and pectin found in fruit and vegetables have more fiber that is completely fermented than do high-cellulose foods, including cereals.[32]

As less fermentable fiber more effectively bulks up stool and adds weight, this may mean added benefits. A meta-analysis of about 100 studies on fiber's effect on stool weight showed that the greater the stool weight, the more dilution of the potentially harmful elements in fecal matter. The various types of dietary fibers differ in the amount they add to fecal weight. For example, 1 gram of wheat bran increases fecal bulk by 5.7 grams, while 1 gram of pectin increases fecal bulk by 1.3 grams.

Also, less fermentable fibers may accelerate the passage of stool through the colon faster than highly fermentable fibers—more efficiently protecting sensitive colon tissues from toxin exposure and other harmful fecal contents.

But some research suggests highly fermentable types of fiber produce more short chain fatty acids than less fermentable fiber. One of these short chain fatty acids, butyrate, may be an anticancer agent, although not all studies on this fatty acid have shown these chemopreventive effects. Several studies indicate that a diet rich in fiber and in fish oil (containing omega-3 fatty acids, which are considered to have anticancer properties) may be more preventive against colon cancer than a high-fiber diet alone.

Thus, consuming fish oil in combination with fiber (highly fermentable or less fermentable) as a bulking agent would benefit health by diluting carcinogens and cancer promoters such as bile acids. The combination of fish oil and fiber may also protect against colon carcinogenesis by inducing cancer cell death.

And so the debate continues on whether dietary fiber can help lower the risk for colorectal cancer. But although fiber's role in cancer reduction has not yet been firmly established, eating plenty of high-fiber foods is still important for good health, as this has been linked to a lower risk of heart disease, diabetes, and other chronic conditions.

TEA AND CANCER PREVENTION

A variety of cell culture and animal model studies indicate that drinking black or green tea (both from the *Camellia sinensis* shrub) may have protective effects against cancer.

Yet the results from epidemiological studies have been inconsistent. Some studies found a link between tea drinking and a reduced risk of cancer, whereas others did not. This contradiction has created uncertainties about tea consumption and its ability to reduce cancer risk.

Studies that show tea's anticancer effects used tea preparations including green tea, black tea (caffeinated and decaffeinated), or total extracts of tea polyphenols. In some cases, researchers used purified green tea compounds (such as epigallocatechin gallate). Most of the studies that used animals switched the animals' drinking water for tea. Tea was also applied directly to skin in a study of skin tumors. Tea appeared to stop tumors from spreading or appearing in these studies.[33]

One hypothesis is that green tea impedes tumor growth by inducing cell death or cell cycle arrest in damaged cells, both protective actions. Also, the antioxidants in green and black teas (including the polyphenols theaflavins and thearubingins) may be chemopreventive agents. Some research has demonstrated that green tea halts activity of phase I enzymes and kick-starts phase II enzymatic action. The balance between the phase I carcinogenic activating enzymes and the phase II detoxifying enzymes could be important in determining the risk for chemically induced cancer.[46,47]

Thus it appears that tea and its polyphenolic compounds may be capable of influencing various enzymes and cellular pathways. Together, these mechanisms may be behind the anticancer effects seen in some research on tea.

Green tea also appeared to help prevent lung cancer in epidemiological studies investigating tea drinking and lung cancer risk among smokers in the United States and Japan. Although smoking is almost twice as common among Japanese men as U.S. men, the rate for lung cancer in Japan is about half of the U.S. rate. Other factors, such as genetic predisposition and lifestyle, may influence this difference in lung cancer risk. Also, the dietary differences between Japan and the United States are considerable, and green tea may be a key factor in this equation. While frequently sipped by most Japanese, it is consumed much less often by most Americans.

However, data from epidemiological studies regarding green tea as a protective factor against lung cancer are somewhat conflicting. Evidence from test-tube studies and animals studies suggest that green tea polyphenols protect against lung cancer,[48,49] while other epidemiological studies of green tea consumption in atomic bomb survivors and postmenopausal women found no association.[50,51] A recent study that investigated green tea drinking and lung cancer in a population-based study found no evidence that green tea reduces lung cancer risk among past or current smokers or those breathing secondhand smoke.[52]

Thus, while it appears that green tea consumption shows benefits in test-tube studies, investigations with humans have not been so supportive. So while some of the results suggest drinking green tea could have profound effects on the molecular and cellular functions as well as health of oral cells in smokers, more studies are needed to back this up. Ultimately, clinical intervention trials should be done to validate the possibly protective mechanisms and actions of tea observed in animal studies.

SUMMARY

While abundant scientific evidence shows that eating plenty of fruit and vegetables lowers cancer risk, it doesn't necessarily follow that taking vitamin supplements can make up for a nutrient shortfall in the diet. Several studies have not found statistically significant benefits from taking vitamin supplements. Worse, in some cases, a high dose may cause cellular damage or other harm, possibly even promoting cancer development.

Population-based studies clearly show that a low risk for cancer is more linked to antioxidant-rich diets featuring generous amounts of vegetables and fruit than to individual dietary antioxidants. This suggests that along with the nutrients in fruit and vegetables other phytonutrients, dietary fiber, or food components may work together, not singly, to offer cancer-prevention benefits.

So a wholesome diet, filled with fruit, vegetables, and fiber appears to be an essential element to cancer prevention. The benefits may even be enhanced with a cup or two of green tea. Or black tea, if that's your preference.

Chapter 22

Controversies Regarding Commonly Perceived Risk Factors and Cancer

New products and technologies can often bring new concerns. Genetically modified foods are a case in point: the debate over the benefits, disadvantages, future implications, and possible risks continues. Some may feel this new ability to mix and match genes is a boon to humankind—others perceive a disaster in the making. While so far no solid evidence links genetically modified foods with cancer, some scientists say it's just too soon to tell.

A few technologies, such as cell phones, seem to consistently cause worry, even when the present evidence shows little or no risk. Other commonly perceived risk factors may be worth avoiding, however. This chapter discusses several points of controversy, including food additives, deodorants, food irradiation, pesticides, and power lines.

GENETICALLY MODIFIED ORGANISMS

Genetically modified organisms (GMOs) are organisms whose genes have been altered (or genetically engineered). In a nutshell, genes from plants, bacteria, viruses, fish, or animals are introduced into an organism's genome to modify the organism to develop, ideally, specific desirable traits. In food crops this could mean resistance to pests, drought, or insecticide. While this could be good news for food production, genetic engineering, particularly of food, has become a heated topic.

Since it was introduced in 1996, the technology has been embraced in some quarters in the United States, and indeed, many U.S. farmers now grow genetically engineered crops. For example, figures from the U.S. Department of Agriculture show that in 2010, 93 percent of the acres in the United States devoted to soybeans were planted with genetically modified herbicide-tolerant soybeans. These soybeans can survive the use of particular herbicides that previously would have killed the crop. Also in 2010, herbicide-tolerant corn was grown on 70 percent of the corn acreage in the United States. These are two of the largest crops, but there are more.[34]

While some scientists celebrate this technology as an answer to world hunger, others are concerned that the host organism's DNA may be affected in negative, unpredictable ways that could eventually harm people. One argument is that all the significant risks that may accompany genetically engineered crops can't possibly be known or anticipated, as the technology is still new—as is science's understanding of genetics. The Union of Concerned Scientists writes,

For example, genetic engineering might be used to produce decaffeinated coffee beans by deleting or turning off genes associated with caffeine production. But caffeine helps protect coffee beans against fungi. Beans that are unable to produce caffeine might be coated with fungi, which can produce toxins. Fungal toxins, such as aflatoxin, are potent human toxins that can remain active through processes of food preparation.[35]

Some scientists are concerned that GMOs may cause disease in people or animals that consume these products in their food. As these genetically engineered foods will be consumed over lifetimes, epidemiological studies may need to be conducted. A European scientific review published in 2009 found that there were few studies examining the safety of genetically modified foods compared to the toxicity studies required for new drugs to be approved. The authors of the review note, "In the absence of adequate safety studies, the lack of evidence that genetically modified food is unsafe cannot be interpreted as proof that it is safe."[36]

This review also found that the use of recombinant growth hormone (recombinant bovine somatotropin, or rBST) in dairy cows to boost milk production should be reexamined as it may promote cancer (although the U.S. Food and Drug Administration approved the animal drug product in 1993 after a safety and efficacy review). Other studies the review analyzed suggest genetically modified foods may have hepatic, pancreatic, renal, and reproductive effects. The review found that genetically engineered food may also influence hematological, biochemical, and immunological systems, the consequences of which are unknown.[36]

Critics note that as natural DNA has been changed in GMOs, the food made with these organisms may affect the human body quite differently from unmodified food, especially with time. Altering the genes in a plant may affect nutrient and antioxidant levels. The long-term effects of a genetically modified diet in humans are simply not known.

A Norwegian study published in 2010 looked at the potential for harm to human health by the consumption of damaged nucleosides as found in digested dietary DNA.[58] The scientists found that a variety of damaged nucleosides "appear to be taken up by cells and incorporated into the cells' own DNA." While most of these damaged nucleosides would be repaired by DNA systems, a small fraction of these could escape repair and eventually create mutations. The study authors suggested this mechanism could contribute to cancer and other diseases in humans, particularly after the consumption of novel foods. The implications from this study suggest that damaged DNA from genetically engineered foods could be incorporated into human DNA. Whether this produces the mutations or cytotoxic effects that lead to cancer requires more investigation and study.

Nevertheless, some scientists write that GMOs in food have been studied much more frequently than traditionally grown and developed food without finding any harmful effects, and thus GMOs are safe and not linked to serious health problems. Some of the literature recommends more research to forestall any unintended consequences, however.[37,38]

Currently, foods that are genetically modified or that contain GMOs are not required to include this information on product labels in the United States.

FOOD ADDITIVES AND CANCER RISK

Many food additives have a popular reputation as carcinogenics, yet the evidence is often lacking. The U.S. Food and Drug Administration maintains a database inventory of more than 3,000 substances it has approved as food additives.[106] Other substances added to food in the United States are not in this list, however, as the FDA has given them approval as generally recognized as safe (GRAS).

The FDA's inventory includes flavor enhancers, artificial sweeteners, colors, anticaking agents (which keep powders free of lumps), preservatives, stabilizers, emulsifiers, humectants, and other food additives that are consumed along with processed foods. Any chemical substance mixed in with food during preparation or storage to achieve a specific effect is a food additive. A discussion follows of some of the more controversial food additives today.

Monosodium Glutamate

The health effects of monosodium glutamate (MSG), a food flavor enhancer, are much discussed but so far no solid evidence links it to cancer. The U.S. Food and Drug Administration classified this additive as a GRAS ingredient but requires MSG to be listed on labels. Well known for its inclusion in some Chinese foods, MSG is also found in processed foods such as sauces, snacks, diet products, packaged meals, salad dressing, cured meats, and canned soups.

Some scientists speculate that MSG may be harmful to human health because the body uses a glutamate derivative as a nerve impulse transmitter in the brain, and MSG's glutamate possibly affects other glutamate-responsive tissues in the body as well. Abnormal function of glutamate receptors has been linked with certain neurological diseases, such as Alzheimer disease and Huntington chorea. Injections of glutamate in laboratory animals have resulted in damage to nerve cells in the brain. Consumption of glutamate in food by laboratory animals, however, does not cause this effect. But published data from studies using animals and humans suggest that MSG consumption is associated with excess weight and other neuroendocrine issues.[65]

Other reports have suggested that MSG use as a food enhancer may cause a type of allergic reaction, the so-called Chinese restaurant syndrome or MSG symptom complex. These symptoms include rapid heartbeat, diarrhea, stomach cramps, flu-like symptoms, depression or mood swings, migraines, dizziness, and panic attacks.

A large multicenter, double-blind, placebo-controlled study in 2000 reported that large doses of MSG given without food may provoke these reactions after MSG-consumption; however, the study noted very low frequency of response from people who identified themselves as symptomatic who ate MSG with food.[66] A review of the scientific literature on the topic in 2006 found that while a general belief persists that MSG causes headache and other symptoms, no consistent clinical data supports this claim.[67]

Thus, recent reviews suggest that in spite of the intense study of MSG, so far no strong scientific information supports the negative effects of MSG on human health in the general population.[68]

Aspartame

Aspartame (sold as Equal or NutraSweet) is an artificial sugar substitute that continues to attract controversy, including cancer fears, long after it was approved by the FDA in 1981. Considered 200 times sweeter than sugar, many food and medical products contain this product, such as instant breakfast foods, breath mints, juice beverages, vitamins, and diet foods.

Aspartame-fed laboratory rats were found to develop lymphomas and leukemias in a 2005 study that caused considerable worry. However, the animals were fed very high doses (the equivalent of 8 to 2,000 cans of diet soda every day) and inconsistencies in the findings were subsequently found, as well as the unexpected result that the cancer rate did not rise with higher doses of the sweetener.[59] Thus, following other studies, the National Cancer Institute, Cancer Research UK, and the European Food Safety Authority have deemed aspartame as safe and not a carcinogen.[103,104,105]

Olestra

Olestra, sold as Olean, is a fat substitute typically found in "light" (or diet) snack foods such as potato chips. While this additive contains zero calories from fat, some people have reported a variety of unpleasant side effects after consumption. These include nausea, cramping, and diarrhea, although various studies including a large clinical trial have not found significant evidence of this.[72,73]

One concern is that olestra may prevent the body's uptake of carotenoids and fat-soluble vitamins, as the fat substitute is neither hydrolyzed by gastrointestinal enzymes nor absorbed.[69] This could have an impact on overall health (depending on the consumption of this additive) as well as the availability of antioxidants to help the body fight diseases such as cancer. Hence, the FDA's approval required that all products with olestra be supplemented with vitamins A, D, E, and K and be labeled to show vitamins had been added to compensate for olestra-related deficits.[70] The FDA removed the labeling requirement in 2003, although the supplemental vitamins are still mandatory.

A recent study found some support for the concern about olestra consumption and serum carotenoids and fat-soluble vitamins. The researchers concluded that olestra was linked with modest but significantly lower circulating carotenoid concentrations, but the fat substitute did not markedly influence serum fat-soluble vitamin concentrations. The researchers suggested that the drop in nutrients would not harm health.[71]

Food Irradiation and DNA Damage

Irradiation of food has sparked concerns that it will damage the nutritive components of food (as it kills most living cells) and make food radioactive or otherwise unsafe to eat.

Manufacturers use ionizing radiation to prevent food-borne illness by destroying microorganisms, bacteria, parasites, or insects and inhibit molds that may be present in food. The technology is less successful at killing viruses and prions (a protein such as the one responsible for mad cow disease, or bovine spongiform encephalopathy) at radiation levels recommended as safe for food. Similar techniques are used to sterilize medical equipment and the food sent with U.S. astronauts into space.[74]

Food poisoning is a significant issue, so this technology could greatly benefit public health. In 2011 about 3,000 people will die because of food-borne disease in the United States, according to figures from the Centers for Disease Control and Prevention (CDC).[75] Another 48 million Americans will get sick, with an estimated 128,000 of them requiring hospitalization for food-borne illnesses. The CDC deems food irradiation as a safe and effective means for reducing food-borne illness, a stand that has been backed up by studies.[74,76]

However, some controversy persists. One study detected the presence of a compound (2-alkylcyclobutanones) found exclusively in irradiated dietary fats that may promote colon carcinogenesis in animals.[77] However, the European Commission's Scientific Committee on Food concluded in July 2002 that genotoxicity of 2-alkylcyclobutanones has not been demonstrated.[78]

Still other studies indicated that irradiation may break down nutrient molecules and destroy the nutritional quality of food. Vitamin B appears to be one of the most sensitive nutrients to radiation, but only small amounts are destroyed.[79]

ENVIRONMENTAL EXPOSURE AND CANCER

As discussed at length in this book, substantial scientific evidence shows lifestyle factors can increase cancer risk, such as smoking tobacco, chronic alcohol abuse, inactivity, excessive sun exposure, obesity, and unhealthy diets. Environmental factors may also play a role in cancer risk, and confusion over concerns as wide-ranging as high-voltage power lines, cell phone use, antiperspirants, and stress may have some people worried that they can't take a step without increasing their chances for a terrible disease.

For example, the worry over deodorants and antiperspirants regarding breast cancer persists despite the lack of evidence suggesting any link.[53] According to Cancer Research UK[54] these concerns began as an e-mail hoax. The debate over the potential risks of power lines is more lively, but it is unlikely that power lines or cell phone use or stress will turn out to be a major cancer risk factor. The section below describes the available scientific evidence that may connect some of these environmental exposures to cancer risk.

Cell Phones and Cancer

No conclusive evidence has tied cell phone use to brain tumors or cancers of the head and neck, according to the National Cancer Institute and numerous studies.[80,81] But as the technology is new and evolving, and because it emits radiofrequency radiation (a type of nonionizing radiation), scientists continue to investigate this topic. The research suggests that not enough radiation is generated by the phones to cause harm (indicated by significant heating of brain tissue or rise in body temperature).

Several epidemiological studies investigated possible links between cell phone use and tumors by comparing patients already diagnosed with tumors with people without brain tumors. Overall, patients with brain tumors did not report higher use of cell phones than the group without tumors.[83]

Given the massive popularity of cell phone use, if the technology was harmful, one might expect to find an increased rate of brain cancer. But this hasn't happened—at least not yet. Some cancers could take decades to develop. Thus parents should perhaps limit their children's access to cell phones, as the youngsters could be at a higher risk for harm due to many years of accumulated exposure. Scientists are also concerned that children may be more vulnerable to harm as they have developing nervous systems that could be more sensitive to radiofrequency radiation.[82] European studies focusing on the risks for children are currently in the works.

So far, one of the largest studies ever to be conducted regarding cell phone use is an international (13 countries) consortium of case-control studies, the INTER-PHONE study, published in 2010.[60] Researchers investigated whether the radiofrequency exposure from cell phone use is linked to a higher risk for cancerous or benign brain tumors and other head and neck tumors. The results showed no evidence for an increased risk for cell phone users, not even for longer call times or for long-time users. However, in 2004 a Swedish study found a slightly higher risk among long-term users for acoustic neuroma, a type of benign brain tumor.[61]

As the evidence regarding cell phone use is still inconclusive, it may be best to keep calls short and limit cell phone use by children.

Power Lines and Cancer

Power lines may be needed for electricity, but they also generate a fair bit of cancer concern due to their electromagnetic fields (EMFs). EMFs are generated by anything that uses or carries electricity, from bedside clock-radios to power lines.

While there is insufficient evidence to show that EMFs pose a cancer risk to adults, some studies have shown a connection between EMFs and a slightly increased risk of childhood leukemia.[84] Scientists with the International Agency for Research on Cancer also found limited evidence that links magnetic fields with childhood leukemia.[110] Other studies, however, have not.[85,64]

In one effort in 2000, researchers gathered data from nine studies from different countries to estimate the leukemia risks for children exposed to power-line EMFs. This research found children had twice the risk of childhood leukemia when exposed to particularly high levels of EMFs.[62] A 2010 follow-up analysis on more recent studies had results similar to the previous pooled analysis, showing an association (although somewhat weaker now) between EMFs and childhood leukemia.[63] It's important to keep in mind that less than 1 percent of children with leukemia come from high-EMF homes.

EMFs may also be responsible for what's called the corona effect: areas of charged particles caught in electric fields that may be inhaled or left on skin. The National Radiological Protection Board in the United Kingdom concluded the effect is real but not likely to be strong enough to cause significant harm.[86]

Stress and Cancer

Studies conducted during the past three decades have found conflicting evidence regarding stress's potential role in cancer. Although some studies have indicated a link between cancer and stress, a direct causal relationship has not been found.[57]

As psychological stress can affect the immune system, which is responsible for fighting infections and diseases such as cancer, it's possible that stress influences cancer development. In dangerous situations a person feels stress, and the body produces stress hormones to help it react to the situation. While small amounts of short-term stress may benefit health, long-term stress may be harmful.

On a physiological level, stress is linked to the increased expression of proinflammatory cytokines, including interleukin 1, interleukin 6, and tumor necrosis factor alpha (TNF-α), and a lowered expression of interleukin 2, interferon, and natural killer cell activity. Most cancers are associated with high levels of TNF-alpha. High levels of TNF-alpha diminish the expression of class I major histocompatibility complex (MHC) antigens on the cell surfaces, thus allowing malignant cells to escape immune surveillance. Therefore stress can promote cancer growth by inhibiting the expression of class I and II MHC molecules and by reducing natural killer cell activity.[87]

Also, stress may lead to cancer indirectly by increasing unhealthy behaviors and habits such as alcohol abuse and overeating and others that cause heart disease. For those people who already have cancer, however, stress could affect tumor growth, according to some studies.[57]

While it is often not possible to avoid some kind of stress, the key to handling the sense of being overwhelmed is to eat nutritious food, get some exercise, be kind, and stay happy.

Deodorants, Antiperspirants, and Cancer

As noted above, no convincing evidence shows a link between these cosmetic products and cancer. The e-mail hoax claimed that antiperspirants stopped the body from sweating out toxins, leading to a toxic buildup in the lymph glands and inducing cancer.[54] Breast cancers, however, don't form that way; they begin in breast tissue and later pass to the lymph glands. Also, a study involving 1,500 women in 2002 found no links between antiperspirant or deodorant use and breast cancer.[53]

In general, the current demand and use of cosmetics such as deodorants may expose people to chemicals with estrogenic or genotoxic properties. Additional investigation of these products and any links to breast cancer may be a good idea.[88]

Pesticides and Cancer

About 20 out of 900 active ingredients in pesticides in the United States have been found to be carcinogenic in animals; not all of the chemicals have been tested.[55]

Agricultural pesticide use has been associated with a variety of cancers, including breast, bowel, leukemia, and lymphoma cancers, according to some studies, although Cancer Research UK deems the current evidence not strong enough for clear answers.[111] An Agricultural Health Study of 300 participants published in 2004 found a possible link between lung cancer in farmers and pesticide use, although follow-up studies were suggested.[56]

In general, people regularly exposed to pesticides, such as farmers and other agricultural workers, are thought to have possibly only a slightly higher risk than the norm for cancer (specifically leukemia and lymphomas) by the International Agency for Research into Cancer.[112] Yet some scientists are concerned that pesticides could suppress the immune system in people regularly exposed to them. A suppressed immune system increases the risk for cancer, but more research is needed to confirm this hypothesis. The current evidence is inconclusive.[89]

Eating fruit and vegetables with minuscule amounts of pesticide is still thought to reduce the risk for cancer, as doses of pesticide chemicals given to laboratory animals tend to be much higher than the amount of pesticides found on fruit and vegetables.[54]

SUMMARY

In discussions of several controversies, this chapter shows a few simple ways to reduce the risk for cancer. For example, taking breaks to relax and lower one's stress may have a beneficial impact on health, over time. And it may reassure some people to know that the biggest health threat regarding cell phone use for adults is when people use the phones while driving—and cause accidents.

Whether to stop eating foods with GMOs or dairy products with bovine growth hormone is another matter. While GMOs are generally recognized as safe, some people may prefer to avoid these products, as the technology is still relatively new. Avoidance may be a challenge, however, as GMOs are not noted on product labels (another topic of much controversy). Pesticides may also be a concern, so shopping for organic foods and local produce might be an answer for a number of people—although vegetables with pesticides have been found to be better for one's health than no vegetables at all.

Finally, while most food additives are deemed safe, it doesn't follow that they should be part of a healthy diet. Ultimately, serving processed foods made with fat and sugar substitutes means less opportunity to eat whole, natural foods that will boost health, well-being, and vitality. And that is not an effective way to fight cancer.

Chapter 23

Conclusion

Cancer has been known as a deadly disease for hundreds of years. Figures from the World Health Organization show that cancer killed more than 7.9 million people in 2010,[5] with the death toll projected to rise to 11 million by 2030.[6] Cancer is a leading cause of death worldwide, although about 30 percent of these deaths are considered preventable. Thus every year, nearly 3 million people might have avoided death, as well as the grief and loss suffered by their families and friends.

While a variety of risk factors may put some people more at risk for cancer than others, ultimately, everyone is at risk for this terrible disease, and the financial and emotional costs are huge. In the United States alone, the National Cancer Institute estimates the overall annual cost for cancer at $107 billion, including $37 billion in direct medical costs, $11 billion in lost productivity, and $59 billion in death costs.[7]

Scientists have been aware for some time that viruses, radiation, and particular chemicals or substances in the environment may promote or trigger cancer. But only recently have researchers learned how normal cells become cancerous. Part of this progress may be credited to the U.S. Congress, after it declared a war on cancer in 1971 and began the investment of billions of dollars into cancer research. One legacy of the push for a cure is a revolutionized understanding of this disease. For example, today we know that, at the cellular level, cancer is a genetic disease and that anything that can damage cell DNA can possibly cause cancer.

Thanks to the efforts and dedication of researchers and health care professionals, new diagnostic tools have been created to help detect early-stage cancer as well as diagnose and treat the disease. This has meant the saving of many lives as well as increased hope and optimism for people who need treatment.

However, in spite of all the research, hard work, and scientific progress, there is still no cure for cancer. Sad news for the more than 4,000 Americans a day who learn they have this disease. But while a cure for cancer is one of the prime goals of research, current progress suggests that the best way to fight cancer is to not get the disease in the first place. In other words, prevention is the key.

CANCER PREVENTION

Some progress has apparently already been made regarding prevention. A November 2008 report from the National Cancer Institute found that, for the first time since records were first kept, in 1971, the overall rates for cancer illness and death in men and women have dropped simultaneously.[8] (The National Cancer Institute records cancer incidence by type, age, sex, and the year of diagnosis for male and female Americans.)

Although overall cancer death rates have been falling for some time now, it's only recently that cancer experts have seen this side-by-side drop in cancer incidence in men and women. The cancers with reduced rates include the three most common cancers in men (lung, colorectal, and prostate) and the two most common cancers in women (colorectal and breast).

The National Cancer Institute report suggests that scientists are making headway in the war against cancer, but these reduced incidence numbers could also indicate that fewer people are undergoing screening for cancer. It could be, for example, that not as many women are having breast cancer screening because health facilities have closed or they no longer have access to testing for some other reason. But because the drop is seen simultaneously in men and women, it is quite possible that prevention efforts are indeed succeeding. The evidence shows that scientific innovation regarding early detection and treatment advances is helping reduce deaths from cancer, yet overwhelming amounts of data support the hypothesis that cancer prevention is the most efficient way to lower cancer rates and death.

Some scientists hypothesize that up to half the cancer deaths in Europe and the United States could be avoided. This is not improbable, as it's known that about a third of all the causes of cancer are from environmental exposures. Many types of cancer are associated with unhealthy lifestyle habits such as smoking tobacco, drinking excessive alcohol, eating a low-nutrient and high-fat diet, and inactivity. Being overweight or obese is also a strong risk factor for a variety of cancers.

But cancer prevention initiatives take time. While tobacco smoke is the single most important risk factor for preventable cancer, it has taken about 40 years for the antismoking public health programs to have an effect on lung cancer rates. Obesity is possibly the next most significant risk factor for preventable cancer, demonstrating the importance of keeping a healthy body weight to avoid cancer. This book is replete with examples of the strong links between exercise (or any regular physical activity) and a reduced risk for breast, colorectal, pancreatic, and prostate cancers. The physical activity needed to lower cancer risk need not be exhaustive; most experts agree that about 30 minutes a day of activities such as gardening, chores, biking, walking, playing sports, or doing housework is sufficient.

Eating a nutritious diet that contains anticancer agents simply involves eating plenty of fruit and vegetables and whole grains. This type of dietary approach has been shown in many studies to be protective against cancer. One example of a healthy dietary approach is the so-called Mediterranean diet, which features a high consumption of vegetables, whole grains, legumes, nuts, fruit, fish, and more monounsaturated fats than saturated fats (as found in meats, particularly red meat). This diet is enhanced with modest amounts of alcohol and low amounts of red meat. Areas where people traditionally eat like this show lower rates of all types of cancer as well as chronic disease such as heart disease. Some scientific experts suggest that poor dietary patterns could be behind as many as 35 percent of all causes of cancer deaths.

Thus, cancer prevention should be the focus of the fight against cancer. Sadly, the prevalence of unhealthy habits in some parts of the world indicates that many people may not know that, in many ways, cancer prevention begins with their choices. Unhealthful dietary habits are often easy to maintain in busy lives and are more accessible (because of the commercialization of junk foods, for example) or may be less expensive and more convenient than eating nutritious foods. Similarly, the urban lifestyle often promotes inactivity. The research shows, however, that, in the long term, exposure to these unhealthy habits can trigger cancer development.

For this reason, cancer prevention should be considered a lifestyle, and people should take all the prevention precautions to better their chances for long healthy lives. Parents should help their children adopt healthy lifestyle habits to lower their overall lifetime cancer risk. This means engaging in regular physical activities and exercise, avoiding tobacco smoke or chronic and excessive alcohol consumption, and eating a nutritious, fruit-and-vegetable-rich diet. Avoiding radiation and numerous chemical exposures (as occur in certain occupations and industries) would also help reduce the risk.

It would be a valuable use of resources if health care systems enhanced cancer prevention awareness through community outreach programs, in addition to cancer screening and treatment. People may also need additional support from their peers and health care professionals when making healthy changes in their lives, such as quitting smoking or losing weight. While regular screening is important for the early detection of cancer (when there is an opportunity for successful treatment), screening itself comes with risks, and doctors should discuss these thoroughly with their patients.

Moreover, the various levels of government could help by establishing public policies that promote and reward exercise and healthy living (such as by making sports or exercise facilities and healthy foods more affordable and accessible).

Likewise, government bodies could impose higher taxes on alcohol and tobacco and even regulate fast foods. Certain food additives and known carcinogens in food preservation should also be banned in the interest of public health. Government agencies have the power to improve public health by imposing regulations to minimize public exposure to known carcinogens, while offering community facilities for safe, accessible physical activity.

CANCER DETECTION

Even if up to half of all cancers are eventually found to be preventable due to lifestyle or environmental exposures (and it's perhaps unrealistic that all the risk factors can be avoided by everyone), many cases of cancer will continue to arise for other reasons. Therefore, while adopting all the advised prevention measures, people should still consult their doctors regarding the recommended screening tests (and the risks of screening) for some of the most common types of cancer. Cancer screening is especially important for people who may be more susceptible to getting a disease because of family history or for those who belong to an ethnic group or have a geographic origin that gives them a disproportionately high risk for cancer.

Recent advances in genetics, particularly as a result of the completion of the Human Genome Project (human DNA sequencing), have improved the detection of mutations and other genetic changes that may play a role in the early stages of cancer development. Scientists can use these biomarkers to find abnormalities that may make people more vulnerable to cancer. Two commonly used genetic tests for cancer include the *BRCA*1 and *BRCA*2 mutations for breast cancer as well as the hereditary nonpolyposis colorectal cancer gene for colorectal cancer. The genetic alterations underlying diseases such as prostate cancer and lung cancer are varied, however, and no main mutation has been noted in either type of cancer.

A technological breakthrough that may help scientists identify specific genetic changes in prostate and lung cancers is DNA or tissue microarray analysis. This technology uses an array of several thousand microscopic spots of DNA oligonucleotide targets. These may be small DNA fragments or short gene segments captured on glass or plastic slides. Probes designed to find specific changes can measure small genetic mutations, such as single nucleotide polymorphisms, chromosomal alterations, and change or loss in gene expression (activity). Through genomewide analysis to find chromosomal regions changed by cancer, this technology is revealing genetic variants that may explain a large proportion of disease in the general population.

For example, scientists have discovered single nucleotide polymorphisms in the human chromosome 8q24 region that influence prostate cancer risk. These mutations are found more often in men of African ancestry than in Caucasians[1] and are likely responsible in part for the disparity seen in prostate cancer rates and death among different ethnic groups. Findings such as this are offering fresh evidence for a causative connection between interindividual genetic variations and human cancer.[2] Other research has found polymorphisms in genes (mannose-binding lectin and the chemokine receptor 5 genes) known to affect susceptibility to bacterial and viral infection. This type of scientific advancement will very probably lead to new genetic biomarkers and, as a result, screening tests for other cancers. Consequently, cancer detection and diagnosis will be improved and some of the fear associated with cancer will be eased.

Yet while the links between these genetic biomarkers and illness have been investigated in depth, little study has been done on how these biomarkers can be applied to predict disease and treatment outcomes. Microarray analysis could be used for genomewide profiling for "fingerprint," or "signature," genes that show variations between normal and cancerous cells and the variations between people. These gene signatures may help reveal the patterns of gene activity in cells that could be tied to disease, as described below.

The Cancer Genome Anatomy Project (CGAP) aims to identify the genes involved in the establishment and growth of human cancer.[9] This research initiative is based on the idea that while every cell contains a full set of the 30,000 human genes, only about 10 percent of them are expressed (active) in any specific cell type. Hence different cell types, such as skin or red blood cells, can be identified via their gene expression pattern. Learning the repertoire of genes expressed in specific cells should result in the fingerprint, or signature, for that type of cell. Researchers expect the signature to change when normal cells become cancerous. For example, there may be an alteration in the expression level of a particular gene in cancerous cells compared to normal cells. With the ability to compare and read these cellular signatures, scientists may be able to create new molecular targets for cancer prevention, detection, and treatment.

The outcome of the CGAP project is expected to revolutionize cancer detection and treatment by allowing these processes to be tailored for individual patients.

A major challenge facing cancer medicine is how to distinguish the diseases that are more likely to develop into invasive cancer from those that will remain largely benign. Following that, scientists aim to separate the patients who would then benefit from treatment after diagnosis from those who would not. The ability to find individual alterations in a cell's signatures, or differentiate between tumors at the molecular level, will improve the sensitivity as well as the specificity of cancer detection.

Already some evidence suggests that gene signatures may improve early detection and lower the risk for lung and breast cancers. Scientists have developed several breast cancer signatures to predict clinical outcomes; these are now being tested in trials (such as the TAILORx).[10] Adding gene signatures for breast cancer to other risk factors or characteristics such as age and tumor size may sharpen predictions of recurrence risk in women with disease in its early stages. It may also help doctors design treatments such as the most effective chemotherapy regimens for breast cancer patients who, following successful treatment, have additional treatment to prevent recurrences.

Researchers can also use this kind of molecular fingerprinting to design new therapies to target specific cellular subtypes of cancer. For example, although patients may have similar kinds of tumors, they may not respond to treatment in the same way. This is due to genetic variances, such as the mutations (known as single nucleotide polymorphisms) seen on the human chromosome 8q24 that are linked to prostate cancer risk. These genetic differences may mean that patients metabolize drugs differently or that particular gene products are present or absent.

In the future, these molecular characteristics could help single out which patients would benefit from a particular type of treatment. So research scientists aim to not only develop new more sensitive and specific tools to discover cancer at its earliest stages but also tailor treatments to each patient. This objective is called personalized medicine.

PERSONALIZED MEDICINE

Researchers believe that in the future doctors will be able to use their patients' individual DNA sequences (genome), or gene expression profiles, to design more personalized treatments, such as the right medicines and doses for each patient's specific needs. This is a relatively new concept in medicine, one that focuses more on the patient than on the disease.[3] This approach will likely improve health outcomes as well as patient experience.

Scientists are already attempting this approach in Florida in a huge project called Total Cancer Care.[11] The project researchers are collecting information such as demographics, clinical profiles, and tumor gene expression profiles from thousands of participating patients. Patients with particular cancer types will receive therapies with drugs that have shown usefulness in respect to their cancer gene expression profile. Because of the large group of participants, many with the same profile could join for early-phase trials with new therapies. This approach may promise better outcomes for these groups than those experienced by patients in the past who participated in previous early-phase trial research.

All of this is thanks to the development of whole genome sequencing and gene expression analysis, which makes it possible to classify each patient according to tumor gene signature pattern. Some of the genes identified as being connected to the diagnosis of cancer are potential biomarkers, not only to identify which patients will benefit from what therapies but also to see if these could be targets themselves for medical treatment. Significantly, this exciting approach in personalized medicine could be used in the treatment and care, and possibly cure, of patients who suffer from diseases other than cancer.

Molecular tests have recently been developed based on the fingerprint signatures linked to breast and colorectal cancers. Soon a lung cancer signature will be available to predict the best treatments for patients. Another promising area is molecular imaging. The new technology aims to combine cell biology and molecular approaches to pick out tumors in the body. The technology employs biosensors to find differences in molecular and biological processes (cell growth rate or cell death, for example) to separate cancer from benign tumors. The result should be improved cancer detection and personalized treatment.

THE FUTURE OF CANCER

New discoveries on clinical, cellular, and molecular levels appear ever more frequently. Scientists seem inspired to work even harder, and so the public can expect significant improvements in cancer screening, diagnosis, and treatment—especially in therapies designed to meet patients' specific needs.

However, the question remains, will there be a cure for cancer?

The answer? Possibly. In some cases, at least. On the basis of our present understanding of this disease, the ongoing scientific and technological advancements should play a large role in the future in significantly reducing cancer incidence and death. Already science, public health, and prevention measures appear to have brought some of these benefits to the United States, as shown by the country's declining cancer rate.

Globally, however, cancer rates are not decreasing. In 2030 about 21 million new cancer cases are expected to be diagnosed, according to the World Health Organization. That same year, 11 million deaths (or 13 million, according to some IARC estimates) due to cancer are also expected. This disturbing trend suggests that cancer rates will have nearly doubled in 20 years and will be the number-one killer in the world, racing past heart disease.[12]

So while Western countries such as the United States appear to be winning the war on cancer, developing countries are experiencing more disease. One factor is that toxic habits from the West are now being embraced in developing countries. Smoking is an excellent example. While public health programs are helping to stop smoking (and limit secondhand smoke exposure) in the United States, Canada, and other Western countries, smoking is increasing elsewhere. Almost half the world's smokers are now people who live in India and China. And smoking rates in these countries are increasing, as they have been for 10 or 15 years. This suggests that, in the next two decades, lung cancer incidence will skyrocket in India and China.

Eventually, the cancer numbers may shift back westward somewhat, because more people than ever before in developed countries are reaching age 70 and older. While this survival rate is good news, as age is an important risk factor for cancer, it also means there will be more people at risk for cancer in the future.

Exciting progress is made in research laboratories and clinics around the world every day. But while we wait for that thrilling moment when the keys for a cure are found, many things can be done to help prevent cancer on an individual level. This book is full of suggestions for preventive measures, such as avoiding cigarette smoke (a major risk factor for lung cancer as well many other diseases), vaccination against hepatitis B to prevent liver cancer (another major cause of death around the world), and human papillomavirus vaccination to prevent cervical cancer (a leading cause of death in women in many areas of South America and Africa). Some ways of eating can protect you from cancer, while other dietary patterns can lead to illness. Governments can play a role, too, in informing the public.[4]

People can take great strides in preventing this devastating disease by adopting the habit of eating five servings of fruit and vegetables daily (or following the so-called Mediterranean diet), ensuring they get regular physical activity, and taking time to relax and enjoy life.

Resources

ORGANIZATIONS

National Cancer Institute (NCI) Cancer Information Service
6116 Executive Boulevard, MSC 8322, Suite 3036A
Bethesda, MD 20892-8322
1-800-4-CANCER
http://cancer.gov
To order NCI publications, visit https://cissecure.nci.nih.gov/ncipubs.

The NCI's Health Informational National Trends Survey (HINTS) Briefs provide snapshots of key data-driven research findings. Visit http://hints.cancer.gov to find population-level estimates regarding specific questions, as well as summaries of significant research findings as a result of analysis on how age, race, and gender influence specific outcomes.

The NCI's State Cancer Legislative Database Program maintains a database of state cancer-related legislation and serves as an important resource for research and analysis of cancer-related health policy. For information about state legislative actions related to cancer prevention, visit http://www.scld-nci.net and select Search Database to access abstracts of more than 5,500 enacted laws and adopted resolutions.

American Cancer Society
1599 Clifton Road, NE
Atlanta, GA 30329
http://www.cancer.org

American Lung Association
61 Broadway, 6th Floor
New York, NY 10006
1-800-586-4872 (1-800-LUNG-USA)
http://www.lungusa.org

Centers for Disease Control and Prevention
4770 Buford Highway, NE
Atlanta, GA 30341-3724.
1-800-311-3435, 1-770-488-5705
http://www.cdc.gov

WEBSITES

National Cancer Institute, A to Z List of Cancers

http://www.cancer.gov/cancertopics/alphalist
Information on more than 50 types of cancer, treatment, screening methods, prevention, statistics, coping with side effects, clinical trials, and more.

National Cancer Institute, Support and Resources

http://www.cancer.gov/cancertopics/support
Support for cancer patients and caregivers, including information on finances, insurance, survivorship, home care, and hospice care, as well as information on managing cancer side effects and complications.

National Cancer Institute, Cancer Topic Searches

http://www.cancer.gov/search/searchcancertopics.aspx
Prepared literature searches of the National Library of Medicine's PubMed database on more than 100 different topics.

Cancer Information Service (CIS)

http://www.cancer.gov/aboutnci/cis
1-800-4-CANCER
Get answers to questions about cancer, smoking cessation assistance, and NCI publications in English and Spanish.

Stand Up to Cancer

http://www.standup2cancer.org
Works to speed innovative cancer research and bring new treatments to patients.

Live Help Online Information Service https://cissecure.nci.nih.gov/livehelp/welcome.asp
Live, online assistance for Web users searching NCI sites.

Smokefree.gov

http://www.smokefree.gov
Offers science-driven tools, information, and support effective in helping smokers quit.

U.S. National Institutes of Health, PubMed

http://www.pubmed.gov
Check scientific publications on cancer and related topics.

Center to Reduce Cancer Health Disparities (CRCHD)

http://crchd.cancer.gov
Offers accurate information for understanding cancer-related inequalities. Provides a monthly e-mail bulletin on cancer health disparities in research, training, and awareness efforts at http://crchd.cancer.gov/news/e-bulletin.html.

Cancer Control PLANET

http://cancercontrolplanet.cancer.gov/
Provides access to data and research-tested resources that can help planners, program staff, and researchers design, implement, and evaluate evidence-based cancer control programs.

FREE OR LOW-COST PUBLICATIONS

American Cancer Society

Publishes a variety of pamphlets and books related to cancer, diet, and lifestyle. To order, visit http://www.cancer.org, call your local chapter of the American Cancer Society, or call 1-800-227-2345.

National Cancer Institute

Publishes a variety of pamphlets and books related to cancer, diet, and lifestyle. Visit http://www.cancer.gov; write to Diet, Nutrition & Cancer Prevention Booklets, National Cancer Institute, Building 31, Room 10A24, Bethesda, MD 20892; or call 1-800-4-CANCER.

Help to quit smoking

To get a free copy of consumer products on quitting smoking, call any of the following toll-free numbers: Agency for Healthcare Research and Quality, 1-800-358-9295; Centers for Disease Control and Prevention, 1-800-CDC-1311; National Cancer Institute, 1-800-4-CANCER or visit the surgeon general's Web site at http://www.surgeongeneral.gov/tobacco.

References

INTRODUCTION

1. Mackay J, Jemal A, Lee NC, Parkin DM. 2006. The history of cancer. *The Cancer Atlas.* American Cancer Society, Atlanta, GA.
2. American Association for Cancer Research. Landmarks in Cancer Research. http://www.aacr.org/home/about-us/centennial/landmarks-in-cancer-research.aspx (accessed Apr. 10, 2011).
3. National Cancer Institute. 2010. Cancer topics: Defining cancer. http://www.cancer.gov/cancertopics/cancerlibrary/what-is-cancer (accessed Apr. 10, 2011).
4. Hanahan D, Weinberg RA. 2000. The hallmarks of cancer. *Cell,* 100, 57–70.
5. Crick F. 1970. Central dogma of molecular biology. *Nature,* 227, 561–3.
6. Alberts B, Bray D, Lewis J, Raff M, Roberts K, Watson JD. 1994. *The Molecular Biology of the Cell.* 3rd ed. New York: Garland Publishing Inc.

CHAPTER 1: BLADDER CANCER

1. Leppert JT, Shvarts O, Kawaoka K, Lieberman R, Belldegrun AS, Pantuck AJ. 2006. Prevention of bladder cancer: a review. *Eur Urol,* 49, 226–34.
2. Cohen SM, Johansson SL. 1992. Epidemiology and etiology of bladder cancer. *Urol Clin North Am,* 19, 421–8.
3. Bjerregaard BK, Raaschou-Nielsen O, Sorensen M, et al. 2006. Tobacco smoke and bladder cancer—in the European Prospective Investigation into Cancer and Nutrition. *Int J Cancer,* 119, 2412–6.
4. Stern MC, Umbach DM, Lunn RM, Taylor JA. 2002. DNA repair gene XRCC3 codon 241 polymorphism, its interaction with smoking and XRCC1 polymorphisms, and bladder cancer risk. *Cancer Epidemiol Biomarkers Prev,* 11, 939–43.
5. Cancer Research UK. 2010. News & resources: Bladder cancer risk factors. http://info.cancerresearchuk.org/cancerstats/types/bladder/riskfactors/ (updated Jun. 25, 2010, accessed Apr. 11, 2011).

6. Chiou HY, Chiou ST, Hsu YH, et al. 2001. Incidence of transitional cell carcinoma and arsenic in drinking water: a follow-up study of 8,102 residents in an arseniasis-endemic area in northeastern Taiwan. *Am J Epidemiol*, 153, 411–8.

7. Geoffroy-Perez B, Cordier S. 2001. Fluid consumption and the risk of bladder cancer: results of a multicenter case-control study. *Int J Cancer*, 93, 880–7.

8. Josephy P D and Mannervik B. 2006. *Molecular toxicology*. 2nd ed. New York: Oxford University Press.

9. National Cancer Institute. Cancer topics: Bladder cancer. http://www.cancer.gov/cancertopics/types/bladder (accessed Apr. 10, 2011).

10. Kogevinas M, 't Mannetje A, Cordier S, et al. 2003. Occupation and bladder cancer among men in Western Europe. *Cancer Cause Control*, 14, 907–14.

CHAPTER 2: BRAIN CANCER

1. McKinney PA. 2005. Central nervous system tumours in children: epidemiology and risk factors. *Bioelectromagnetics*, Suppl 7, S60–S68.

2. Farrell CJ, Plotkin SR. 2007. Genetic causes of brain tumors: neurofibromatosis, tuberous sclerosis, von Hippel-Lindau, and other syndromes. *Neurol Clin*, 25, 925–46.

3. Alexander V. 1991. Brain tumor risk among United States nuclear workers. *Occup Med*, 6, 695–714.

4. Davis FS. 2007. Epidemiology of brain tumors. *Expert Rev Anticancer Ther*, 7 (suppl), S3–S6.

5. Huang K, Whelan EA, Ruder AM, et al. 2004. Reproductive factors and risk of glioma in women. *Cancer Epidemiol Biomarkers Prev*, 13, 1583–8.

6. McKinley BP, Michalek AM, Fenstermaker RA, Plunkett RJ. 2000. The impact of age and sex on the incidence of glial tumors in New York State from 1976 to 1995. *J Neurosurg*, 93, 932–9.

7. Kley N, Whaley J, Seizinger BR. 1995. Neurofibromatosis type 2 and von Hippel-Lindau disease: from gene cloning to function. *Glia*, 15, 297–307.

8. Reuss D, von Deimling A. 2009. Hereditary tumor syndromes and gliomas. *Recent Results Cancer Res*, 171, 83–102.

9. Wrensch M, Weinberg A, Wiencke J, et al. 1997. Does prior infection with varicella-zoster virus influence risk of adult glioma? *Am J Epidemiol*, 145, 594–7.

10. Poltermann S, Schlehofer B, Steindorf K, Schnitzler P, Geletneky K, Schlehofer JR. 2006. Lack of association of herpesviruses with brain tumors. *J Neurovirol*, 12, 90–9.

11. Aboulafia DM, Ratner L, Miles SA, Harrington WJ Jr. 2006. Antiviral and immunomodulatory treatment for AIDS-related primary central nervous system lymphoma: AIDS Malignancies Consortium pilot study 019. *Clin Lymphoma Myeloma*, 6, 399–402.

12. Wrensch M, Minn Y, Chew T, Bondy M, Berger MS. 2002. Epidemiology of primary brain tumors: current concepts and review of the literature. *Neuro Oncol*, 4, 278–99.

13. National Brain Tumor Society. Tumor types. http://www.braintumor.org/patients-family-friends/about-brain-tumors/tumor-types/ (accessed Apr. 10, 2011).

14. Ha M, Im H, Lee M, et al. 2007. Radio-frequency radiation exposure from AM radio transmitters and childhood leukemia and brain cancer. *Am J Epidemiol*, 166, 270–9.

15. Preston DL, Ron E, Yonehara S, et al. 2002. Tumors of the nervous system and pituitary gland associated with atomic bomb radiation exposure. *J Natl Cancer Inst,* 94, 1555–63.

16. Silvera SA, Miller AB, Rohan TE. 2006. Hormonal and reproductive factors and risk of glioma: a prospective cohort study. *Internal J Cancer,* 118, 1321–4.

17. Bachinski LL, Olufemi S, Zhou X, et al. 2005. Genetic mapping of a third Li-Fraumeni syndrome predisposition locus to human chromosome 1q23. *Cancer Res,* 65, 427–431.

18. Grant R, Ironside JW. 1995. Glutathione S-transferase and cytochrome P450 detoxifying enzyme distribution in human cerebral glioma. *J Neuro Oncol,* 25, 1–7.

19. Bondy ML, Wang, LE, El-Zein R, et al. 2001. Gamma-radiation sensitivity and risk of glioma. *J Natl Cancer Inst,* 93, 1553–7.

20. Blot WJ, Henderson BE, Boice JD Jr. 1999. Childhood cancer in relation to cured meat intake: review of the epidemiological evidence. *Nutr Cancer,* 34, 111–8.

21. McCredie M, Maisonneuve P, Boyle P. 1994. Perinatal and early postnatal risk factors for malignant brain tumors in New South Wales children. *Int J Cancer,* 56, 11–15.

22. Bluhm EC, Zahm SH, Fine HA, et al. 2007. Personal hair dye use and risks of glioma, meningioma, and acoustic neuroma among adults. *Am J Epidemiol,* 65, 63–71.

23. Davis JR, Brownson RC, Garcia R, et al. 1993. Family pesticide use and childhood brain cancer. *Arch Environ Contam Toxicol,* 24, 87–92.

CHAPTER 3: BREAST CANCER

1. Key T, Appleby P, Barnes I, Reeves G. 2002. Endogenous sex hormones and breast cancer in postmenopausal women: reanalysis of nine prospective studies. *J Natl Cancer Inst,* 94, 606–16.

2. Erlandsson G, Montgomery SM, Cnattingius S, Ekbom A. 2003. Abortions and breast cancer: record-based case-control study. *Int J Cancer,* 103, 676–9.

3. Land CE, Tokunaga M, Koyama K, et al. 2003. Incidence of female breast cancer among atomic bomb survivors, Hiroshima and Nagasaki, 1950–1990. *Radiat Res,* 160, 707–17.

4. Wolff MS, Weston A. 1997. Breast cancer risk and environmental exposures. *Environ Health Perspect,* 105 (suppl 4), 891–6.

5. Kaufman DJ, Beaty TH, Struewing JP. 2003. Segregation analysis of 231 Ashkenazi Jewish families for evidence of additional breast cancer susceptibility genes. *Cancer Epidemiol Biomarkers Prev,* 12, 1045–52.

6. Evans JP, Skrzynia C, Susswein L, Harlan M. 2005–2006.Genetics and the young woman with breast cancer. *Breast Dis,* 23, 17–29.

7. Tarone RE and Chu KC. 2002. The greater impact of menopause on ER- than ER+ breast cancer incidence: a possible explanation (United States). *Cancer Causes Control,* 13, 7–14.

8. Ghafoor A, Jemal A, Ward E, Cokkinides V, Smith R, Thun M. 2003. Trends in breast cancer by race and ethnicity. *CA Cancer J Clin,* 53, 342–55.

9. Sellers TA, Kushi LH, Cerhan JR, et al. 2001. Dietary folate intake, alcohol, and risk of breast cancer in a prospective study of postmenopausal women. *Epidemiology,* 12, 420–8.

10. Brinton LA, Sherman ME, Carreon JD, Anderson WR. 2008. Recent trends in breast cancer among younger women in the United States. *J Natl Cancer Inst,* 100, 1477–81.
11. Stark A, Kleer CG, Martin I, et al. 2010. African ancestry and higher prevalence of triple negative breast cancer findings from an international study. *Cancer,* 116, 4926–32.
12. Pinheiro SP, Holmes MD, Pollak MN, et al. 2005. Racial differences in premenopausal endogenous hormones. *Cancer Epidemiol Biomarkers Prev,* 14, 2147–53.
13. Peters TM, Schatzkin A, Gierach GL. 2009. Physical activity and postmenopausal breast cancer risk in the NIH-AARP diet and health study. *Cancer Epidemiol Biomarkers Prev,* 18, 289–96.
14. Holm LE, Callmer E, Hjalmer ML, et al. 1989. Dietary habits and prognostic factors in breast cancer. *JNCI,* 81,1218–23.
15. Conlon MS, Johnson KC, Bewick MA, et al. 2010. Smoking (active and passive), *N*-acetyltransferase 2 and risk of breast cancer. *Cancer Epi,* 34, 142–9.
16. National Cancer Institute. Cancer topics: Breast cancer. http://www.cancer.gov/cancertopics/types/breast (accessed Apr. 10, 2011).

CHAPTER 4: CERVICAL CANCER

1. Wright TC Jr, Schiffman M. 2003. Adding a test for human papillomavirus DNA to cervical-cancer screening. *N Engl J Med,* 348, 489–90.
2. Winer RL, Lee SK, Hughes JP, Adam DE, Kiviat NB, Koutsky LA. 2003. Genital human papillomavirus infection: incidence and risk factors in a cohort of female university students. *Am J Epidemiol,* 157, 218–26.
3. Rigoni S. 1987. Statistical facts about cancers on which Doctor Rigoni-Stern based his contribution to the Surgeons' Subgroup of the IV Congress of the Italian Scientists on 23 September 1842. (translation). *Stat Med,* 6, 881–4.
4. Scheffner M, Munger K, Byrne JC, Howley PM. 1991. The state of the p53 and retinoblastoma genes in human cervical carcinoma cell lines. *Proc Natl Acad Sci USA,* 88, 5523–7.
5. Cymet TC. 2006. Sexually activated or transmitted? Questions about HPV. *J Am Osteopath Assoc,* 106, 423.
6. Haverkos HW. 2004. Viruses, chemicals and co-carcinogenesis. *Oncogene,* 23, 6492–9.
7. Prokopczyk B, Cox JE, Hoffmann D, Waggoner SE. 1997. Identification of tobacco-specific carcinogen in the cervical mucus of smokers and nonsmokers. *J Natl Cancer Inst,* 89, 868–73.
8. Baldwin A, Huh KW, Munger K. 2006. Human papillomavirus E7 oncoprotein dysregulates steroid receptor coactivator 1 localization and function. *J Virol,* 80, 6669–77.
9. Hernandez BY, McDuffie K, Zhu X, et al. 2005. Anal human papillomavirus infection in women and its relationship with cervical infection. *Cancer Epidemiol Biomarkers Prev,* 14, 2550–6.
10. Leyden WA, Manos MM, Geiger AM, et al. 2005. Cervical cancer in women with comprehensive health care access: attributable factors in the screening process. *J Natl Cancer Inst,* 97, 675–83.

11. Cox JT. 2006. Epidemiology and natural history of HPV. *J Fam Pract,* November (suppl), 3–9 Review.
12. Cason J, Rice P, Best JM. 1998. Transmission of cervical cancer-associated human papilloma virus from mother to child. *Intervirology,* 44, 213–8.
13. Haverkos HW. 2005. Multifactorial etiology of cervical cancer: a hypothesis. *MedGenMed,* 7(4), 57.
14. Clarke EA, Anderson TW. 1979. Does screening by "PAP" smears help prevent cervical cancer? A case-control study. *Lancet,* 314, 1–4.
15. Lee M, Lin T-L, Horne DA. 2009. FDA statistical review and evaluation Gardasil efficacy. http://www.fda.gov/downloads/BiologicsBloodVaccines/Vaccines/ApprovedProducts/UCM190978.pdf (accessed Apr. 12, 2011).
16. GLOBOCAN. 2008. Cancer incidence and mortality. Prediction. World cervix uteri. http://globocan.iarc.fr/burden.asp?selection_pop=220900&Text-p=World&selection_cancer=4152&Text-c=Cervix+uteri&pYear=2&type=1&window=1&submit=%A0Execute%A0 (accessed Apr. 10, 2011).

CHAPTER 5: COLORECTAL CANCER

1. Potter JD. 1999. Colorectal cancer: molecules and populations. *J Natl Cancer Inst,* 91, 916–32.
2. Narayan S, Roy D. 2003. Role of APC and DNA mismatch repair genes in the development of colorectal cancers. *Mol Cancer,* 2, 41.
3. Umar A, Kunkel TA. 1996. DNA-replication fidelity, mismatch repair and genome instability in cancer cells. *Eur J Biochem,* 238, 297–307.
4. Campos FG, Logullo Waitzberg AG, Kiss DR, Waitzberg DL, Habr-Gama A, Gama-Rodrigues J. 2005. Diet and colorectal cancer: current evidence for etiology and prevention. *Nutr Hosp,* 20, 18–25.
5. Hamer HM, Jonkers D, Venema K, Vanhoutvin S, Troost FJ, Brummer RJ. 2008. Review article: the role of butyrate on colonic function. *Aliment Pharmacol Ther,* 27, 104–19.
6. Peters U, Chatterjee N, McGlynn KA, et al. 2004. Calcium intake and colorectal adenoma in a U.S. colorectal cancer early detection program. *Am J Clin Nutr,* 80, 1358–65.
7. Hardman AE. 2001. Physical activity and cancer risk. *Proc Nutr Soc,* 60, 107–13.
8. Giovannucci E. 2001. An updated review of the epidemiological evidence that cigarette smoking increases risk of colorectal cancer. *Cancer Epidemiol Biomarkers Prev,* 10, 725–31.
9. National Cancer Institute. 2010. Cancer topics: What you need to know about cancer of the colon and rectum. http://www.cancer.gov/cancertopics/wyntk/colon-and-rectal/page1 (accessed Apr. 2011).
10. Center MM, Jemal A, Smith RA, Ward E. 2009. Worldwide variations in colorectal cancer. *CA Cancer J Clin,* 59, 366–78.
11. Bandipalliam P. 2005. Syndrome of early onset colon cancers hematologic malignancies and feature of neurofibromatosis in HNPCC families with homozygous mismatch repair gene mutation. *Familial Cancer,* 4, 323–3.
12. Seitz HK, Maurer B, Stickel F. 2005. Alcohol consumption and cancer of the gastrointestinal tract. *Dig Dis,* 23, 297–303.

13. National Cancer Institute. 2010. Cancer topics: Colon and rectal cancer. http://www. cancer.gov/cancertopics/types/colon-and-rectal (accessed Apr. 9, 2011).
14. Goldman R and Shields PG. 2003. Food mutagens. *J Nutr.* 133 Suppl 3, 965S–73S.

CHAPTER 6: ESOPHAGEAL CANCER

1. Gao Y, Hu N, Han X, et al. 2009. Family history of cancer and risk for esophageal and gastric cancer in Shanxi, China. *BMC Cancer,* 9, 269.
2. Engel LS, Chow WH, Vaughan TL, et al. 2003. Population attributable risks of esophageal and gastric cancers. *J Natl Cancer Inst,* 95, 1404–13.
3. Souza RF, Spechler SJ. 2005. Concepts in the prevention of adenocarcinoma of the distal esophagus and proximal stomach. *CA Cancer J Clin,* 55, 334–51.
4. Risk JM, Mills HS, Garde J, et al. 1999. The tylosis esophageal cancer (TOC) locus: more than just a familial cancer gene. *Dis Esophagus,* 12, 173–6.
5. Hiyama T, Yoshihara M, Tanaka S, Chayama K. 2007. Genetic polymorphisms and esophageal cancer risk. *Int J Cancer,* 121, 1643–58.
6. Yu Y, Taylor PR, Li JY, et al. 1993. Retrospective cohort study of risk-factors for esophageal cancer in Linxian, People's Republic of China. *Cancer Causes Control,* 4, 195–202.
7. Blot WJ, Li JY, Taylor PR, et al. 1993. Nutrition intervention trials in Linxian, China: supplementation with specific vitamin/mineral combinations, cancer incidence, and disease-specific mortality in the general population. *J Natl Cancer Inst,* 85, 1483–92.
8. Yokoyama A, Muramatsu T, Ohmori T, Higuchi S, Hayashida M, Ishii H. 1996. Esophageal cancer and aldehyde dehydrogenase-2 genotypes in Japanese males. *Cancer Epidemiol Biomarkers Prev,* 5, 99–102.
9. Ghavamzadeh A, Moussavi A, Jahani M, Rastegarpanah M, Iravani M. 2001. Esophageal cancer in Iran. *Semin Oncol,* 28, 153–7.
10. Castellsague X, Munoz N, De SE, Victora CG, Castelletto R, Rolon PA. 2000. Influence of mate drinking, hot beverages and diet on esophageal cancer risk in South America. *Int J Cancer,* 88, 658–64.
11. World Health Organization, IARC, GLOBOCAN. 2008, Cancer incidence and mortality worldwide (prediction for esophageal cancer in 2010). http://globocan.iarc.fr/burden.asp?selection_pop=220900&Text-p=World&selection_cancer=19040&Text-c=Oes ophagus&pYear=2&type=1&window=1&submit=%A0Execute%A0 (accessed Apr. 9, 2011).
12. Kamangar F, Malekzadek R, Dawsey SM, et al. 2007. Esophageal cancer in northeastern Iran: a review. *Arch Iranian Med,* 10, 70–82.
13. Tryhus MR, Davis M, Griffith JK, et al. 1989. Familial achalasia in twin siblings: significance of possible hereditary role. *J Pediatric Surg,* 24, 292–5.
14. Goode EL, Ulrich CM, Potter JD. 2002. Polymorphisms in DNA repair genes and associations with cancer risk. *Cancer Epidemiol Biomarkers Prev,* 11, 1513–30.
15. Newberne PM. 1985. Dietary factors affecting biological responses to esophageal and colon chemical carcinogens. In: *Xenobiotic Metabolism: Nutritional Effects.* ACS Symposium Series, American Chemical Society; Vol. 277, Chapter 13, pp. 163–76.

16. Pandeya N, Williams G, Green AC, Webb PM, Whiteman DC. 2009. Alcohol consumption and the risk of adenocarcinoma and squamous cell cancer of esophagus, *Gastroenterology,* 136, 1155–7.

17. Lee J-M, Liu TY, et al. 2005. Safrole-DNA adducts in tissues from esophageal cancer patients: clues to areca-related esophageal carcinogenesis. *Mutat Res,* 565, 121–8.

18. Wei WQ, Abnet CC, Lu N, Roth MJ, Wang GQ, Dye BA, Dong ZW, Taylor PR, Albert P, Qiau YL, Dawsey SM. 2005. Risk factors for esophageal squamous dysplasia in adult inhabitants of a high risk region of China. *Gut,* 54, 759–63.

19. National Cancer Institute. Cancer topics: Esophageal cancer. http://www.cancer.gov/cancertopics/types/esophageal (accessed Apr. 8, 2011).

20. Munitiz V, Parrilla P, Ortiz A, Matinez-de-Haro L, Yelamos J, Molina J. 2008. High risk of malignancy- familial Barrett's esophagus: Presentation of one family. *J of Clin Gastroenterolog.* 42, 806–9.

21. Chu FS, Li GY. 1994. Simultaneous occurrence of fumonisin B-1 and other mycotoxins in mouldy corn collected from the Peoples Republic of China in regions with high incidences of esophageal cancer. *Appl Environ Microbiol.* 60, 847–52.

22. Makun HA, Anjorin ST, Moronfoye B, Adejo FO, Afolabi OA, Fagbayibo G, et al. 2010. Fungal and aflatoxin contamination of some human food commodities in Nigeria. *Afr J Food Sci.* 4, 127–35.

CHAPTER 7: GASTRIC CANCER

1. Graham S, Haughey B, Marshall J, et al. 1990. Diet in the epidemiology of gastric cancer. *Nutr Cancer,* 13, 19–34.

2. Alexander GA, Brawley OW. 2000. Association of Helicobacter pylori infection with gastric cancer. *Mil Med,* 165, 21–7.

3. Suzuki S, Muroishi Y, Nakanishi I, Oda Y. 2004. Relationship between genetic polymorphisms of drug-metabolizing enzymes (CYP1A1, CYP2E1, GSTM1, and NAT2), drinking habits, histological subtypes, and p53 gene point mutations in Japanese patients with gastric cancer. *J Gastroenterol,* 39, 220–30.

4. Farthing MJ, Fitzgerald R, Zhang ZW. 2001. Acid, helicobacter and immunity: a new paradigm for oesophagogastric cancer. *J Physiol Paris,* 95, 423–7.

5. Mayne ST, Risch HA, Dubrow R, et al. 2001. Nutrient intake and risk of subtypes of esophageal and gastric cancer. *Cancer Epidemiol Biomarkers Prev,* 10, 1055–62.

6. National Cancer Institute. 2010. Cancer topics: Stomach (gastric) cancer. http://www.cancer.gov/cancertopics/types/stomach (accessed Apr. 9, 2010).

7. El-Omar EM, Carrington M, Chow WH, et al. 2000. Interleukin-1 polymorphisms associated with increase risk of gastric cancer. *Nature,* 404, 398–402.

8. Figueiredo C, Machado JC, Pharoah P, et al. 2002. Helicobacter pylori and interluekin I genotyping: an opportunity to identify high-risk individuals for gastric carcinoma. *J Natl Cancer Inst,* 94, 1680–7.

9. Navarro Silvera SA, Mayne ST, Risch H, et al. 2008. Food group intake and risk of subtype of esophageal and gastric cancer. *Int J Cancer,* 123, 852–60.

CHAPTER 8: HEAD AND NECK CANCER

1. Slotman GJ, Swaminathan AP, Rush BF Jr. 1983. Head and neck cancer in a young age group: High incidence in black patients. *Head Neck Surg,* 5, 293–8.
2. Ye H, Yu T, Temam S, et al. 2008. Transcriptomic dissection of tongue squamous cell carcinoma. *BMC Genomics,* 9, 69.
3. Johnson N. 2001. Tobacco use and oral cancer: A global perspective. *J Dent Educ,* 65, 328–39.
4. Ragin CC, Modugno F, Gollin SM. 2007. The epidemiology and risk factors of head and neck cancer: a focus on human papillomavirus. *J Dent Res,* 86, 104–14.
5. Hashibe M, Brennan P, Benhamou S, et al. 2007. Alcohol drinking in never users of tobacco, cigarette smoking in never drinkers, and the risk of head and neck cancer: pooled analysis in the International Head and Neck Cancer Epidemiology Consortium. *J Natl Cancer Inst,* 99, 777–89.
6. Wang Y, Spitz MR, Lee JJ, Huang M, Lippman SM, Wu X. 2007. Nucleotide excision repair pathway genes and oral premalignant lesions. *Clin Cancer Res,* 13, 3753–8.
7. An J, Liu Z, Hu Z, et al. 2007. Potentially functional single nucleotide polymorphisms in the core nucleotide excision repair genes and risk of squamous cell carcinoma of the head and neck. *Cancer Epidemiol Biomarkers Prev,* 16, 1633–8.
8. Chen K, Hu Z, Wang LE, et al. 2007. Polymorphic TP53BP1 and TP53 gene interactions associated with risk of squamous cell carcinoma of the head and neck. *Clin Cancer Res,* 13, 4300–5.
9. Rossi M, Garavello W, Talamini R, et al. 2007. Flavonoids and the risk of oral and pharyngeal cancer: a case-control study from Italy. *Cancer Epidemiol Biomarkers Prev,* 16, 1621–5.
10. Wen X, Walle T. 2005. Preferential induction of CYP1B1 by benzo[a]pyrene in human oral epithelial cells: impact on DNA adduct formation and prevention by polyphenols. *Carcinogenesis,* 26, 1774–81.
11. Morse DE, Psoter WJ, Cleveland D, et al. 2007. Smoking and drinking in relation to oral cancer and oral epithelial dysplasia. *Cancer Causes Control,* 18, 919–29.
12. Kabat GC, Wynder EL. 1989. Type of alcoholic beverage and oral cancer. *Int J Cancer,* 43, 190–4.
13. Visapaa JP, Gotte K, Benesova M, et al. 2004. Increased cancer risk in heavy drinkers with the alcohol dehydrogenase 1C*1 allele, possibly due to salivary acetaldehyde. *Gut,* 53, 871–6.
14. Chen YC, Hunter DJ. 2005. Molecular epidemiology of cancer. *CA Cancer J Clin,* 55, 45–54.
15. Tezal M, Sullivan MA, Reid M E, et al. 2007. Chronic periodontitis and the risk of tongue cancer. *Arch Otolaryngol Head Neck Surg,* 133, 450–4.
16. Shavers VL, Harlan LC, Winn D, Davis WW. 2003. Racial/ethnic patterns of care for cancers of the oral cavity, pharynx, larynx, sinuses, and salivary glands. *Cancer Metastasis Rev,* 22, 25–38.
17. National Cancer Institute. 2010. SEER (Surveillance Epidemiology and End Results) data, stat fact sheet: Oral cavity and pharynx. http://www.seer.cancer.gov/statfacts/html/oralcav.html (accessed March 27, 2011).

18. Egeli U, Ozkan L, Tunca B, et al. 2000. The relationship between genetic susceptibility to head and neck cancer with the expression of common fragile sites. *Head Neck,* 22, 591–8.

19. Reshmi S, Cand Gollin SM. 2005. Chromosomal instability in oral cancer cells. *J Dent Res,* 84, 107–17.

20. World Health Organization, IARC, GLOBOCAN Project. 2008. Cancer incidence and mortality worldwide in 2008 (with online analysis/prediction tables for future years) http://globocan.iarc.fr/ (accessed Apr. 9, 2011).

CHAPTER 9: LEUKEMIA AND LYMPHOMA

1. Legler JM, Ries LA, Smith MA, et al. 1999. Cancer surveillance series [corrected]: brain and other central nervous system cancers: Recent trends in incidence and mortality. *J Natl Cancer Inst,* 91, 1382–90.

2. Goldman M. 1982. Ionizing radiation and its risks. *West J Med,* 137, 540–7.

3. Belson M, Kingsley B, Holmes A. 2007. Risk factors for acute leukemia in children: a review. *Environ Health Perspect,* 115, 138–45.

4. Descatha A, Jenabian A, Conso F, Ameille J. 2005. Occupational exposures and haematological malignancies: overview on human recent data. *Cancer Causes Control,* 16, 939–53.

5. Morrissette JJ, Halligan GE, Punnett HH, McKenzie AS, Guerrero F, de Chadarevian JP. 2006. Down syndrome with low hypodiploidy in precursor B-cell acute lymphoblastic leukemia. *Cancer Genet Cytogenet,* 169, 58–61.

6. Chang JS, Selvin S, Metayer C, Crouse V, Golembesky A, Buffler PA. 2006. Parental smoking and the risk of childhood leukemia. *Am J Epidemiol,* 163, 1091–100.

7. Tang D, Warburton D, Tannenbaum SR, et al. 1999. Molecular and genetic damage from environmental tobacco smoke in young children. *Cancer Epidemiol Biomarkers Prev,* 8, 427–31.

8. Fraga CG, Motchnik PA, Wyrobek AJ, Rempel DM, Ames BN. 1996. Smoking and low antioxidant levels increase oxidative damage to sperm DNA. *Mutat Res,* 351, 199–203.

9. Rauscher GH, Sandler DP, Poole C, et al. 2003. Is family history of breast cancer a marker of susceptibility to exposures in the incidence of de novo adult acute leukemia? *Cancer Epidemiol Biomarkers Prev,* 12, 289–94.

10. Grulich AE, Wan X, Law MG, et al. 2000. B-cell stimulation and prolonged immune deficiency are risk factors for non-Hodgkin's lymphoma in people with AIDS. *AIDS,* 14, 133–40.

11. Cannon M, Cesarman E. 2000. Kaposi's sarcoma-associated herpes virus and acquired immunodeficiency syndrome-related malignancy. *Semin Oncol,* 27, 409–19.

12. Grulich AE, Vajdic CM, Cozen W. 2007. Altered immunity as a risk factor for non-Hodgkin lymphoma. *Cancer Epidemiol Biomarkers Prev,* 16, 405–8.

13. Chang ET, Smedby KE, Hjalgrim H, et al. 2005. Family history of hematopoietic malignancy and risk of lymphoma. *J Natl Cancer Inst,* 97, 1466–74.

14. Landgren O, Zhang Y, Zahm SH, Inskip P, Zheng T, Baris D. 2006. Risk of multiple myeloma following medication use and medical conditions: a case-control study in Connecticut women. *Cancer Epidemiol Biomarkers Prev,* 15, 2342–7.

15. Folley JH, Borges W, Yamawaki T. 1952. Incidence of leukemia in survivors of the atomic bomb in Hiroshima and Nagasaki, Japan. *Am J Med*, 13, 311–21.
16. Archer VE. 1987. Association of nuclear fallout with leukemia in the United States. *Arch Environ Health*, 42, 263–71.
17. Cantor KP, Strickland PT, Brock JW, et al. 2003. Risk of non-Hodgkin's lymphoma and prediagnostic serum organchlorines. *Environ Health Perspective*, 111, 179–83.
18. George ED, Sadovsky R. 1999. Multiple myeloma: Recognition and management. *Am Fam Physician*, 59, 185–94.
19. Rubinsten MA. 1949. Multiple myeloma as a form of leukemia. *Blood*, 4, 1049–67.
20. Ries LAG, Eisner MP, Kosary CL et al. 2003. SEER cancer statistics review, 1975–2000. Bethesda, MD. National Cancer Institute.
21. Lewis DR, Pottern LM, Brown LM, et al. 1994. Multiple myeloma among blacks and whites in the United States: The role of chronic antigenic stimulation. *Cancer Causes Control*, 5, 2547–54.
22. National Cancer Institute. 2010. Cancer topics: Leukemia. http://www.cancer.gov/cancertopics/types/leukemia (accessed Apr. 9, 2011).
23. National Cancer Institute. 2010. Cancer topics: Hodgkin lymphoma. http://www.cancer.gov/cancertopics/types/hodgkin (accessed Apr. 9, 2011).
24. National Cancer Institute. 2010. Cancer topics: Non-Hodgkin lymphoma. http://www.cancer.gov/cancertopics/types/non-hodgkin (accessed Apr. 9, 2011).

CHAPTER 10: LIVER CANCER

1. Veldt BJ, Chen W, Heathcote EJ, et al. 2008. Increased risk of hepatocellular carcinoma among patients with hepatitis C cirrhosis and diabetes mellitus. *Hepatology*, 47, 1856–62.
2. Gurtsevitch VE. 2008. Human oncogenic viruses: Hepatitis B and hepatitis C viruses and their role in hepatocarcinogenesis. *Biochemistry (Mosc)*, 73, 504–13.
3. Yamanaka T, Shiraki K, Nakazaawa S, et al. 2001. Impact of hepatitis B and C virus infection on the clinical prognosis of alcoholic liver cirrhosis. *Anticancer Res*, 21, 2937–40.
4. Peers FG, Linsell CA. 1973. Dietary aflatoxins and liver cancer-a population based study in Kenya. *Br J Cancer*, 27, 473–84.
5. Budhu A, Wang XW. 2006. The role of cytokines in hepatocellular carcinoma. *J Leukoc Biol*, 80, 1197–213.
6. Yu MC, Yuan JM. 2004. Environmental factors and risk for hepatocellular carcinoma. *Gastroenterology*, 127 (suppl 1), S72–S78.
7. Turner PC, Sylla A, Diallo MS, Castegnaro JJ, Hall AJ, Wild CP. 2002. The role of aflatoxins and hepatitis viruses in the etiopathogenesis of hepatocellular carcinoma: A basis for primary prevention in Guinea-Conakry, West Africa. *J Gastroenterol Hepatol*, 17 (suppl), S441–S448.
8. Teufel A, Staib F, Kanzler S, Weinmann A, Schulze-Bergkamen H, Galle PR. 2007. Genetics of hepatocellular carcinoma. *World J Gastroenterol*, 13, 2271–82.
9. Jackson PE, Qian GS, Friesen MD, et al. 2001. Specific p53 mutations detected in plasma and tumors of hepatocellular carcinoma patients by electrospray ionization mass spectrometry. *Cancer Res*, 61, 33–5.

10. Inoue M, Yoshimi I, Sobue T, Tsugane S. 2005. Influence of coffee drinking on subsequent risk of hepatocellular carcinoma: a prospective study in Japan. *J Natl Cancer Inst*, 97, 293–300.
11. Gish RG. 2007. Improving outcomes for patients with chronic hepatitis B 19. *Hepatol Res*, 37 (suppl 1), S67–S78.
12. World Health Organization. 2011. Global alert and response, Hepatitis B. http://www.who.int/csr/disease/hepatitis/whocdscsrlyo20022/en/index1.html (accessed Apr. 9, 2011).
13. Richelle M, Tavazzi I, Offord E. 2001. Comparison of the antioxidant activity of commonly consumed polyphenolic beverages (coffee, cocoa, and tea) prepared per cup serving. *J Agric Food Chem*, 49, 3438–42.
14. National Academy of Sciences. 2009. The hepatitis B story. http://www.beyonddiscovery.org/content/view.article.asp?a=265 (accessed Apr. 9, 2011).
15. International Agency for Research on Cancer; GLOBOCAN. 2008. Liver cancer incidence and mortality worldwide in 2008. http://globocan.iarc.fr/factsheets/cancers/liver.asp (accessed Apr. 9, 2011).
16. International Agency for Research on Cancer; GLOBOCAN. 2008. Prediction. World cancer estimations for 2008 and 2010. http://globocan.iarc.fr/burden.asp?selection_pop=220900&Text-p=World&selection_cancer=13070&Text-c=Liver&pYear=2&type=0&window=1&submit=%A0Execute%A0 (accessed Apr. 9, 2011).
17. National Cancer Institute. 2010. Cancer topics: Liver cancer. http://www.cancer.gov/cancertopics/types/liver (accessed Apr. 9, 2011).

CHAPTER 11: LUNG CANCER

1. Doll R, Hill AB. 1950. Smoking and carcinoma of the lung: preliminary report. *Br Med J*, 2, 739–48.
2. Leischow SJ, Djordjevic MV. 2004. Smoking reduction and tobacco-related cancers: the more things change, the more they stay the same. *J Natl Cancer Inst*, 96, 86–7.
3. Jones SC, Travers MJ, Hahn EJ, et al. 2006. Secondhand smoke and indoor public spaces in Paducah, Kentucky. *J Ky Med Assoc*, 104, 281–8.
4. Subramanian J, Govindan R. 2007. Lung cancer in never smokers: a review. *J Clin Oncol*, 25, 561–70.
5. Benowitz NL. 1992. Cigarette smoking and nicotine addiction. *Med Clin North Am*, 76, 415–37.
6. Moody PM. 1984. Human smoking patterns and smoke deliveries. *Int J Addict*, 19, 431–9.
7. Woo RS, Park EY, Shin MS, et al. 2002. Mechanism of nicotine-evoked release of 3H-noradrenaline in human cerebral cortex slices. *Br J Pharmacol*, 137, 1063–70.
8. Frankish HM, Dryden S, Wang Q, Bing C, MacFarlane IA, Williams G. 1995. Nicotine administration reduces neuropeptide Y and neuropeptide Y mRNA concentrations in the rat hypothalamus: NPY may mediate nicotine's effects on energy balance. *Brain Res*, 694, 139–46.
9. Cohen C, Pickworth WB, Henningfield JE. 1991. Cigarette smoking and addiction. *Clin Chest Med*, 12, 701–10.
10. Brunnemann KD, Hoffmann D. 1991. Analytical studies on tobacco-specific N-nitrosamines in tobacco and tobacco smoke. *Crit Rev Toxicol*, 21, 235–40.

11. Rabinoff M, Caskey N, Rissling A, Park C. 2007. Pharmacological and chemical effects of cigarette additives. *Am J Public Health,* 97, 1981–91.
12. Willems EW, Rambali B, Vleeming W, Opperhuizen A, van Amsterdam JG. 2006. Significance of ammonium compounds on nicotine exposure to cigarette smokers. *Food Chem Toxicol,* 44, 678–88.
13. Keithly L, Ferris WG, Cullen DM, Connolly GN. 2005. Industry research on the use and effects of levulinic acid: a case study in cigarette additives. *Nicotine Tob Res,* 7, 761–71.
14. Ezzati M, Lopez AD. 2003. Measuring the accumulated hazards of smoking: global and regional estimates for 2000. *Tobacco Control,* 12, 79–85.
15. Pfeifer GP, Denissenko MF, Olivier M, Tretyakova N, Hecht SS, Hainaut P. 2002. Tobacco smoke carcinogens, DNA damage and p53 mutations in smoking-associated cancers. *Oncogene,* 21, 7435–51.
16. Rickert WS, Robinson JC, Bray DF, Rogers B, Collishaw NE. 1985. Characterization of tobacco products: a comparative study of the tar, nicotine, and carbon monoxide yields of cigars, manufactured cigarettes, and cigarettes made from fine-cut tobacco. *Prev Med,* 14, 226–33.
17. Muller FH. 1939. Tobacco use and lung carcinoma. *Z Krebsforsch,* 49, 57.
18. Berthiller J, Sasco AJ. 2005. Smoking (active or passive) in relation to fertility, medically assisted procreation and pregnancy. *J Gynecol Obstet Biol Reprod (Paris),* 1, 3547–54.
19. Tobacco-Free Kids: The Role of Tobacco in the United States. http://www.tobacco-freekids.org/facts_issues/toll_us/ (accessed Apr. 9, 2011).
20. Baker F, Ainsworth SR, et al. 2000. Health risks associated with cigar smoking. *JAMA,* 284, 735–40.
21. National Cancer Institute. Tobacco Control Research. http://cancercontrol.cancer.gov/tcrb/monographs/20/index.html (accessed Apr. 9, 2011).
22. Liu P, Vikis HG, Lu Y, Wang Y, et al. 2010. Cumulative effect of multiple loci on genetic susceptibility to familial lung cancer. *Cancer Epidemiol Biomarkers Prev,* 19, 517–24.
23. National Cancer Institute. 2010. Cancer topics: Lung cancer. http://www.cancer.gov/cancertopics/types/lung (accessed Apr. 9, 2011).
24. Bailey-Wilson JE, Amos CI, Pinney SM, Peterson GM, de Andrade M, et al. 2004. A major lung cancer susceptibility locus maps to chromosome 6q23-25. *Am J Hum Genet,* 75, 460–74.
25. National Cancer Institute. 2010. Cancer topics: Smoking: Tobacco facts. http://www.cancer.gov/cancertopics/tobacco/smoking (accessed Apr. 9, 2011).

CHAPTER 12: OVARIAN AND ENDOMETRIAL CANCERS

1. Lubin F, Chetrit A, Modan B, Freedman LS. 2006. Dietary intake changes and their association with ovarian cancer risk. *J Nutr,* 136, 2362–7.
2. Kushi LH, Mink PJ, Folsom AR, et al. 1999. Prospective study of diet and ovarian cancer. *Am J Epidemiol,* 149, 21–31.
3. Larsson SC, Holmberg L, Wolk A. 2004. Fruit and vegetable consumption in relation to ovarian cancer incidence: the Swedish Mammography Cohort. *Br J Cancer,* 90, 2167–70.

4. Seeger H, Wallwiener D, Kraemer E, Mueck AO. 2005. Estradiol metabolites are potent mitogenic substances for human ovarian cancer cells. *Eur J Gynaecol Oncol,* 26, 383–5.

5. Lancaster JM, Sayer RA, Blanchette C, et al. 2006. High expression of insulin-like growth factor binding protein-2 messenger RNA in epithelial ovarian cancers produces elevated preoperative serum levels. *Int J Gynecol Cancer,* 16, 1529–35.

6. Tworoger SS, Lee IM, Buring JE, Pollak MN, Hankinson SE. 2007. Insulin-like growth factors and ovarian cancer risk: a nested case-control study in three cohorts. *Cancer Epidemiol Biomarkers Prev,* 16, 1691–5.

7. Schmeler KM, Lynch HT, Chen LM, et al. 2006. Prophylactic surgery to reduce the risk of gynecologic cancers in the Lynch syndrome. *N Engl J Med,* 354, 261–9.

8. Holschneider CH, Berek JS. 2000. Ovarian cancer: epidemiology, biology and prognostic factors. *Semin Surg Oncol,* 19, 3–10.

9. Purdie DM, Bain CJ, Siskind V, et al. 2003. Ovulation and risk of epithelial ovarian cancer. *Int J Cancer,* 104, 228–32.

10. National Cancer Institute. 2010. Cancer topics: Endometrial cancer. http://www.cancer.gov/cancertopics/types/endometrial (accessed December 2010).

11. Ciernikova S, Tomka M, Kovac M, et al. 2006. Ashkenazi founder BRCA1/BRCA2 mutations in Slovak hereditary breast and/or ovarian cancer families. *Neoplasma,* 53, 97–102.

12. Levine DA, Lin O, Barakat RR, et al. 2001. Risk of endometrial carcinoma associated with BRCA mutation. *Gynecol Oncol,* 80, 395–8.

13. Preston DL, Ron E, Tokuoka S, et al. 2007. Solid cancer incidence in atomic bomb survivors: 1958–1998. *Radiation Res,* 168, 1–64.

14. Preston DL, Shimizu Y, Pierce DA. 2003. Studies of mortality of atomic bomb survivors. *Radiation Res,* 160, 381–407.

15. Melin A, Sparen P. 2007. The risk of cancer and the role of parity among women with endometrosis. *Human Reprod,* 22, i27–i28.

16. National Cancer Institute. 2010. Cancer topics: Ovarian cancer. http://www.cancer.gov/cancertopics/types/ovarian (accessed Apr. 7, 2011).

CHAPTER 13: PANCREATIC CANCER

1. Michaud DS. 2004. Epidemiology of pancreatic cancer. *Minerva Chir,* 59, 99–111.

2. Michaud DS, Giovannucci E, Willett WC, Colditz GA, Stampfer MJ, Fuchs CS. 2001. Physical activity, obesity, height, and the risk of pancreatic cancer. *JAMA,* 286, 921–9.

3. Muscat JE, Stellman SD, Hoffmann D, Wynder EL. 1997. Smoking and pancreatic cancer in men and women. *Cancer Epidemiol Biomarkers Prev,* 6, 15–19.

4. Klein AP, Brune KA, Petersen GM, et al. 2004. Prospective risk of pancreatic cancer in familial pancreatic cancer kindreds. *Cancer Res,* 64, 2634–8.

5. Lowenfels AB, Maisonneuve P, Lankisch PG. 1999. Chronic pancreatitis and other risk factors for pancreatic cancer. *Gastroenterol Clin North Am,* 28, 673–85

6. Uygur-Bayramicli O, Dabak R, Orbay E, et al. 2007. Type 2 diabetes mellitus and CA 19–9 levels. *World J Gastroenterol,* 13, 5357–9.

7. Larsson SC, Bergkvist L, Wolk A. 2006. Consumption of sugar and sugar-sweetened foods and the risk of pancreatic cancer in a prospective study. *Am J Clin Nutr,* 84, 1171–6.

8. Alguacil J, Porta M, Benavides FG, et al. 2000. Occupation and pancreatic cancer in Spain: a case-control study based on job titles. PANKRAS II Study Group. *Int J Epidemiol,* 29, 1004–13.

9. Risch HA. 2003. Etiology of pancreatic cancer, with a hypothesis concerning the role of N-nitroso compounds and excess gastric acidity. *J Natl Cancer Inst,* 95, 948–60.

10. Anderson KE, Sinha R, Kulldorff M, et al. 2002. Meat intake and cooking techniques: associations with pancreatic cancer. *Mutat Res,* 506, 225–31.

11. Gallicchio L, Kouzis A, Genkinger JM, et al. 2006. Active cigarette smoking, household passive smoke exposure, and the risk of developing pancreatic cancer. *Prev Med,* 42, 200–5.

12. Hasan MM, Abbruzzese JL, Bondy ML, Wolff RA, et al. 2007. Passive smoking and the use of noncigarette tobacco products in association with risk for pancreatic cancer: a case-control study. *Cancer,* 109, 2547–56.

13. Li D, Xie K, Wolff R, Abbruzzese JL. 2004. Pancreatic cancer. *Lancet,* 363, 1049–57.

14. Pezzilli R, Casadei R, Morselli-Labate AM. 2009. Is type 2 diabetes a risk factor for pancreatic cancer? *JOP. J Pancreas,* 10(6), 705–6.

15. International Agency for Research on Cancer; GLOBOCAN. 2008. Cancer incidence and mortality worldwide. World predictions for pancreatic cancer, 2010. http://globocan.iarc.fr/burden.asp?selection_pop=220900&Text-p=World&selection_cancer=22090&Text-c=Pancreas&pYear=2&type=1&window=1&submit=%A0Exec ute%A0 (accessed Apr. 7, 2011).

16. National Cancer Institute. 2010. Cancer topics: Pancreatic cancer. http://www.cancer.gov/cancertopics/types/pancreatic (accessed Apr. 13, 2011).

CHAPTER 14: PROSTATE CANCER

1. De Marzo AM, Meeker AK, Zha S, et al. 2003. Human prostate cancer precursors and pathobiology. *Urology,* 62 (suppl 1), 55–62.

2. Kwabi-Addo B, Chung W, Shen L, et al. 2007. Age-related DNA methylation changes in normal human prostate tissues. *Clin Cancer Res,* 13, 3796–802.

3. Zeegers MP, Kiemeney LA, Nieder AM, Ostrer H. 2004. How strong is the association between CAG and GGN repeat length polymorphisms in the androgen receptor gene and prostate cancer risk? *Cancer Epidemiol Biomarkers Prev,* 13 (pt 1), 1765–71.

4. Palapattu GS, Sutcliffe S, Bastian PJ, et al. 2005. Prostate carcinogenesis and inflammation: emerging insights. *Carcinogenesis,* 26, 1170–81.

5. Platz EA, Rimm EB, Willett WC, Kantoff PW, Giovannucci E. 2000. Racial variation in prostate cancer incidence and in hormonal system markers among male health professionals. *J Natl Cancer Inst,* 92, 2009–17.

6. Gann PH, Hennekens CH, Ma J, Longcope C, Stampfer MJ. 1996. Prospective study of sex hormone levels and risk of prostate cancer. *J Natl Cancer Inst,* 88, 1118–26.

7. De Marzo AM, Platz EA, Sutcliffe S, et al. 2007. Inflammation in prostate carcinogenesis. *Nat Rev Cancer,* 7, 256–69.

8. Huang WY, Hayes R, Pfeiffer R, et al. 2008. Sexually transmissible infections and prostate cancer risk. *Cancer Epidemiol Biomarkers Prev,* 17, 2374–81.

9. Alcaraz A, Hammerer P, Tubaro A, Schroder FH, Castro R. 2009. Is there evidence of a relationship between benign prostatic hyperplasia and prostate cancer? Findings of a literature review. *Eur Urol,* 55, 864–73.

10. Ehrlichman RJ, Isaacs JT, Coffey DS. 1981. Differences in the effects of estradiol on dihydrotestosterone induced prostate growth of the castrated dog and rat. *Invest Urol,* 18, 466–70.

11. Mahapokai W, Xue Y, van Garderen E, et al. 2000. Cell kinetics and differentiation after hormonal-induced prostatic hyperplasia in the dog. *Prostate,* 44, 40–8.

12. Asamoto M, Hokaiwado N, Cho YM, et al. 2001. Prostate carcinomas developing in transgenic rats with SV40 T antigen expression under probasin promoter control are strictly androgen dependent. *Cancer Res,* 61, 4693–700.

13. Jackson MA, Kovi J, Heshmat MY, et al. 1980 Characterization of prostatic carcinoma among blacks: a comparison between a low-incidence area, Ibadan, Nigeria, and a high-incidence area, Washington DC. *Prostate,* 1, 185–205.

14. Odedina FT, Akinremi TO, Chinegwundoh F, Roberts R, et al. 2009 Prostate cancer disparities in Black men of African descent: a comparative literature review of prostate cancer burden among Black men in the United States, Caribbean, United Kingdom, and West Africa. *Infect Agents Cancer,* 4 (suppl 1), S2.

15. Gudmundsson J, Sulem P, Manolescu A, et al. 2007. Genome-wide association study identifies a second prostate cancer susceptibility variant at 8q24. *Nat Genet,* 39, 631–7.

16. National Cancer Institute. 2010. Cancer topics: Prostate cancer. http://www.cancer. gov/cancertopics/types/prostate (accessed Apr. 7, 2011).

CHAPTER 15: SKIN CANCER

1. National Center for Health Statistics, National Cancer Institute. 2010. SEER stat fact sheets: Melanoma of the skin. http://seer.cancer.gov/statfacts/html/melan.html (accessed Apr. 9, 2011).

2. Daya-Grosjean L, Sarasin A. 2005. The role of UV induced lesions in skin carcinogenesis: an overview of oncogene and tumor suppressor gene modifications in xeroderma pigmentosum skin tumors. *Mutat Res,* 571, 43–56.

3. Wilson LD, Housman D, Smith BD. 2005. Merkel cell carcinoma: improved outcome with the addition of adjuvant therapy. *J Clin Oncol,* 23, 7236–7.

4. National Cancer Institute. 2010. Fact sheet: Cryosurgery in cancer treatment: Questions and answers. http://www.cancer.gov/cancertopics/factsheet/Therapy/cryosurgery (accessed Apr. 13, 2011).

5. Gorlin RJ. 1995. Nevoid basal cell carcinoma syndrome. *Dermatol Clin,* 13, 113–25.

6. Iftner A, Klug SJ, Garbe C, et al. 2003. The prevalence of human papillomavirus genotypes in nonmelanoma skin cancers of nonimmunosuppressed individuals identifies high-risk genital types as possible risk factors. *Cancer Res,* 63, 7515–9.

7. Curtin JA, Fridlyand J, Kageshita T, et al. 2005. Distinct sets of genetic alterations in melanoma. *N Engl J Med,* 353, 2135–47.

8. Fears TR, Guerry D, Pfeiffer RM, et al. 2006. Identifying individuals at high risk of melanoma: a practical predictor of absolute risk. *J Clin Oncol,* 24, 3590–6.

9. Roewert-Huber J, Stockfleth E, Kerl H. 2007. Pathology and pathobiology of actinic (solar) keratosis—an update. *Br J Dermatol,* 157 (suppl 2), 18–20.
10. Staberg B, Wulf HC, Poulsen T, Klemp P, Brodthagen H. 1983. Carcinogenic effect of sequential artificial sunlight and UV-A irradiation in hairless mice. Consequences for solarium "therapy." *Arch Dermatol,* 119, 641–3.
11. Bolshakov S, Walker CM, Strom SS, Selvan Ms, Clayman GL, El-Naggar A, et al. 2003. p53 mutations in human aggressive and nonaggressive basal and squamous cell carcinomas. *Clin. Cancer Res,* 9, 228–34.
12. Yang X, Pfeiffer RM, Goldstein AM. 2006. Influence of glutathione-S-transferase (GSTMI, GSTPI, GSTTI) and Cytochrome p450 (CYPIAi, CYP2D6) polymorphisms on numbers of basal cell carcinomas. *J Med Genet,* 43, e16.
13. Woo DK, Eide MJ. 2010. Tanning beds, skin cancer and vitamin D: an examination of the scientific evidence and public health implications. *Dermatol Ther,* 23, 61–71.
14. Berwick M. 2008. Are tanning beds "safe"? Human studies of melanoma. *Pigment Cell Melanoma Res,* 21, 517–9.
15. Feng H, Shuda M, Chang Y and Moore P. 2008 Clonal integration of a polyomavirus in human Merkel cell carcinoma. *Science,* 319(5866), 1096–1100.
16. U.S. Environmental Protection Agency. 2010. SunWise program. Skin cancer facts. http://www.epa.gov/sunwise/background.html (accessed Mar. 16, 2011).

CHAPTER 16: OCCUPATION-ASSOCIATED CANCER

1. Waldron HA. 1983. A brief history of scrotal cancer. *Br J Ind Med,* 40, 390–401.
2. Siemiatycki J, Richardson L, Straif K, et al. 2004. Listing occupational carcinogens. *Environ Health Perspect,* 112, 1447–59.
3. Blair A, Rothman N, Zahm SH. 1999. Occupational cancer epidemiology in the coming decades. *Scand J Work Environ Health,* 25, 491–7.
4. Boffetta P. 2004. Epidemiology of environmental and occupational cancer. *Oncogene,* 23, 6392–403.
5. Baker DB, Landrigan PJ. 1990. Occupationally related disorders. *Med Clin North AM,* 74(2), 441–60.
6. Tola S. 1980. Occupational cancer of the urinary bladder. *J Toxicol Environ Health,* 6(5–6), 1253–60.
7. Gottschall EB. 2002. Occupational and environmental thoracic malignancies. *J Thorac Imaging,* 17(3), 189–97.
8. Bruske-Hohlfeld I. 2009. Environmental and occupational risk factors for lung cancer. *Methods Mol Biol,* 472, 3–23.
9. Sathia Kumar N, Delzell E, Amoateng-Adjepong Y, et al. 1997. Epidemiologic evidence on the relationship between mists containing sulfuric acid and respiratory track cancer. *Crit Rev Toxicol,* 27, 233–51.
10. Kuntz HD, May B. 1980. Occupational liver diseases [in German]. *MMW Munch Med Wochenschr,* 122, 1059–62.
11. Gawkrodger DJ. 2004. Occupational skin cancers. *Occup Med (Lond),* 54, 458–63.
12. Khalade A, Jaakkola MS, Pukkala E, Jaakkola JJ. 2010. Exposure to benzene at work and the risk of leukemia: a systemic review and meta-analysis. *Environ Health,* 9, 31. http://www.cancer.gov/newsletter/cancer-and-the environment.

CHAPTER 17: NUTRITION AND CANCER

1. Michels KB. 2003. Nutritional epidemiology—past, present, future. *Int J Epidemiol,* 32, 486–8.
2. Doll R, Peto R. 1981. The causes of cancer: Quantitative estimates of avoidable risks of cancer in the United States today. *J Natl Cancer Inst,* 66, 1191–308.
3. Trichopoulou A, Costacou T, Bamia C, Trichopoulos D. 2003. Adherence to a Mediterranean diet and survival in a Greek population. *N Engl J Med,* 348, 2599–608.
4. Foran JA, Carpenter DO, Hamilton MC, Knuth BA, Schwager SJ. 2005. Risk-based consumption advice for farmed Atlantic and wild Pacific salmon contaminated with dioxins and dioxin-like compounds. *Environ Health Perspect,* 113, 552–6.
5. Sinha R, Peters U, Cross AJ, et al. 2005. Meat, meat cooking methods and preservation, and risk for colorectal adenoma. *Cancer Res,* 65, 8034–41.
6. Ryan BM, Weir DG. 2001. Relevance of folate metabolism in the pathogenesis of colorectal cancer. *J Lab Clin Med,* 138, 164–76.
7. Kushi L, Giovannucci E. 2002. Dietary fat and cancer. *Am J Med,* 113 (suppl 9B), 63S–70S.
8. Curtin K, Bigler J, Slattery ML, Caan B, Potter JD, Ulrich CM. 2004. MTHFR C677T and A1298C polymorphisms: diet, estrogen, and risk of colon cancer. *Cancer Epidemiol Biomarkers Prev,* 13, 285–92.
9. Chen J, Stampfer MJ, Hough HL, et al. 1998. A prospective study of N-acetyltransferase genotype, red meat intake, and risk of colorectal cancer. *Cancer Res,* 58, 3307–11.
10. Fleischauer AT, Arab L. 2001. Garlic and cancer: a critical review of the epidemiologic literature. *J Nutr,* 131 (suppl), 1032S–40S.
11. Campbell JK, Canene-Adams K, Lindshield BL, Boileau TW, Clinton S. K., Erdman JW Jr. 2004. Tomato phytochemicals and prostate cancer risk 4. *J Nutr,* 134 (suppl), 3486S–92S.
12. Hammami I, Amara S, Benahmed M, El May MV, Mauduit C. 2009. Chronic crude garlic-feeding modified adult male rat testicular markers: mechanisms of action. *Reprod Biol Endocrinol,* 7, 65.
13. Fleischauer AT, Poole C, Arab L. 2000. Garlic consumption and cancer prevention: meta-analyses of colorectal and stomach cancers. *Am J Clin Nutr,* 72, 1047–52.
14. Arora DS, Kaur J. 1999. Antimicrobial activity of spices. *Int J Antimicrob Agents,* 12, 257–62.
15. Singh SV, Srivastava SK, Choi S, et al. 2005. Sulforaphane-induced cell death in human prostate cancer cells is initiated by reactive oxygen species. *J Biol Chem,* 280, 19911–24.
16. Hecht SS. 1999. Chemoprevention of cancer by isothiocyanates, modifiers of carcinogen metabolism. *J Nutr,* 129, 768S–74S.
17. Hakim IA, Harris RB, Brown S, et al. 2003. Effect of increased tea consumption on oxidative DNA damage among smokers: a randomized controlled study. *J Nutr,* 133 (suppl), 3303S–9S.
18. Fritz WA, Eltoum IE, Cotroneo MS, Lamartiniere CA. 2002. Genistein alters growth but is not toxic to the rat prostate. *J Nutr,* 132, 3007–11.
19. Zhou JR, Yu L, Mai Z, Blackburn GL. 2004. Combined inhibition of estrogen-dependent human breast carcinoma by soy and tea bioactive components in mice. *Int J Cancer,* 108, 8–14.

20. Venkateswaran V, Fleshner NE, Sugar LM, Klotz LH. 2004. Antioxidants block prostate cancer in lady transgenic mice. *Cancer Res,* 64, 5891–6.

21. Milner JA. 2004. Molecular targets for bioactive food components. *J Nutr,* 134 (suppl), 2492S–8S.

22. Pokharel YR, Han EH, Kim J, Oh SJ, et al. 2006. Potent protective effect of isoimperatorin against aflatoxin B_1-inducible cytotoxicity in H4IIE cells: bifunctional effects on glutathione *S*-transferase and CYP_{1A}. *Carcinogenesis,* 27, 2483–90.

23. Cho YA, Kim J, Park KS, Lim SY, et al. 2010. Effect of dietary soy intake on breast cancer risk according to menopause and hormone receptor status. *Eur J Clin Nutr,* 64, 924–32.

24. Wu AH, Yu MC, Tseng C-C, et al. 2009. Dietary patterns and breast cancer risk in Asian American women. *Am J Clin Nutr,* 89, 1145–54.

25. Lau TY, Lueg LK. 2006. Soya isoflavones suppress phorbal 12-myristate-13-acetate-induced cOX-2 expression in MCF-7 cells. *Br J Nutr,* 96, 169–76.

26. Navarro-Alarion M, Cabrera-Vique C. 2008. Selenium in food and the human body: a review. *Sci Total Environ,* 400, 115–41.

27. Liu X, Allen JD, Arnold JT, and Blackburn MR. 2008. Lycopene inhibits IGF-1 signal transduction and growth in normal prostate epithelial cells by decreasing DHT-modulated IGF-1 production in co-cultured reactive stromal cells. *Carcinogenesis,* 29, 816–23.

28. National Institutes of Health, Office of Dietary Supplements. 2011. Dietary supplement fact sheet: Vitamin D. http://ods.od.nih.gov/factsheets/vitamind (accessed Apr. 7, 2011).

29. National Institutes of Health, Office of Dietary Supplements. 2009. Dietary supplement fact sheet: Selenium. http://ods.od.nih.gov/factsheets/selenium/ (accessed Apr. 7, 2011).

30. Peters U, Chatterjee N, Church TR, Mayo O, Sturup S, Foster CB, et al. 2006. High serum selenium and reduced risk of advanced colorectal adenoma in a colorectal cancer early detection program. *Cancer Epidemiol Biomarkers Prev,* 15, 315–20.

CHAPTER 18: BODY WEIGHT AND CANCER

1. Calle EE, Rodriguez C, Walker-Thurmond K, Thun MJ. 2003. Overweight, obesity, and mortality from cancer in a prospectively studied cohort of U.S. adults. *N Engl J Med,* 348, 1625–38.

2. Levine JA. 2004. Non-exercise activity thermogenesis (NEAT). *Nutr Rev,* 62 (suppl), S82–S97.

3. Wellman NS, Friedberg B. 2002. Causes and consequences of adult obesity: health, social and economic impacts in the United States. *Asia Pac J Clin Nutr,* 11 (suppl), S705–S709.

4. Kennedy GC. 1953. The role of depot fat in the hypothalamic control of food intake in the rat. *Proc R Soc Lond B Biol Sci,* 140, 578–96.

5. Gibbs J, Young RC, Smith GP. 1973. Cholecystokinin decreases food intake in rats. *J Comp Physiol Psychol,* 84, 488–95.

6. Schwartz MW, Woods SC, Porte D Jr, Seeley RJ, Baskin DG. 2000. Central nervous system control of food intake. *Nature,* 404, 661–71.

7. Barsh GS, Schwartz MW. 2002. Genetic approaches to studying energy balance: perception and integration. *Nat Rev Genet,* 3, 589–600.

8. Campfield LA, Smith FJ, Burn P. 1998. Strategies and potential molecular targets for obesity treatment. *Science,* 280, 1383–7.
9. Wilson BD, Ollmann MM, Barsh GS. 1999. The role of agouti-related protein in regulating body weight. *Mol Med Today,* 5, 250–6.
10. Hofbauer KG. 2002. Molecular pathways to obesity. *Int J Obes Relat Metab Disord,* 26 (suppl), S18–S27.
11. Drewnowski A. 2004. Obesity and the food environment: dietary energy density and diet costs. *Am J Prev Med,* 27 (suppl), 154–62.
12. Friedenreich CM, Orenstein MR. 2002. Physical activity and cancer prevention: etiologic evidence and biological mechanisms. *J Nutr,* 132 (suppl), 3456S–64S.
13. Hursting SD, Lavigne JA, Berrigan D, et al. 2004. Diet-gene interactions in p53-deficient mice: insulin-like growth factor-1 as a mechanistic target. *J Nutr,* 134 (suppl), 2482S–6S.
14. Mahabir S, Baer DJ, Johnson LL, et al. 2006. Usefulness of body mass index as a sufficient adiposity measurement for sex hormone concentration associations in postmenopausal women. *Cancer Epidemiol Biomarkers Prev,* 15, 2502–7.
15. Wang Y, Jacobs EJ, Patel AV, et al. 2008. A prospective study of waist circumference and body mass index in relation to colorectal cancer incidence. *Cancer Causes Control,* 19, 783–92.
16. Wellen KE, Hotamisligil GS. 2005. Inflammation, stress, and diabetes. *J Clin Invest,* 115, 1111–9.
17. Hursting SD, Perkins SN, Brown CC, Haines DC, Phang JM. 1997. Calorie restriction induces a p53-independent delay of spontaneous carcinogenesis in p53-deficient and wild-type mice. *Cancer Res,* 57, 2843–6.
18. Bult MJ, van Dalen T, Muller AF. 2008. Surgical treatment of obesity. *Eur J Endocrinol,* 158, 135–45.
19. Mito N, Yoshino H, Hosoda T, Sato K. 2004. Analysis of the effect of leptin on immune function in vivo using diet-induced obese mice. *J Endocrinol,* 180, 167–73.
20. Pelleymounter MA. 1997. Leptin and the physiology of obesity. *Current Pharmaceutical Design,* 3, 85–98.
21. Ashizawa N, Yahata T, Quan J, Adachi S, Yoshihawa K and Tanaka K. 2010. Serum leptin-adiponectin ratio and endometrial cancer risk in postmenopausal female subjects. *Gynecologic Oncology,* 119, 65–69.

CHAPTER 19: IMMUNE SYSTEM AND CANCER RISK

1. Chaplin DD. 2003. 1. Overview of the immune response. *J Allergy Clin Immunol,* 111 (suppl), S442–S459.
2. Madsen BE, Ramos EM, Boulard M, et al. 2008. Germline mutation in RNASEL predicts increased risk of head and neck, uterine cervix and breast cancer. *PLoS One,* 3, e2492.
3. Lan Q, Zheng T, Rothman N, et al. 2006. Cytokine polymorphisms in the Th1/Th2 pathway and susceptibility to non-Hodgkin lymphoma. *Blood,* 107, 4101–8.
4. Sharma RA, Browning MJ. 2005. Mechanisms of the self/non-self-survey in the defense against cancer: potential for chemoprevention? *Crit Rev Oncol Hematol,* 56, 5–22.
5. Lin WW, Karin M. 2007. A cytokine-mediated link between innate immunity, inflammation, and cancer. *J Clin Invest,* 117, 1175–83.

6. Bernig T, Boersma BJ, Howe TM, et al. 2007. The mannose-binding lectin (MBL2) haplotype and breast cancer: an association study in African-American and Caucasian women. *Carcinogenesis,* 28, 828–36.
7. Stockbrugger RW. 1999. Nonsteroidal anti-inflammatory drugs (NSAIDs) in the prevention of colorectal cancer. *Eur J Cancer Prev,* 8 (suppl), S21–S25.
8. Chew BP, Park JS. 2004. Carotenoid action on the immune response. *J Nutr,* 134 (suppl), 257S–61S.
9. Xue L, Pestka JJ, Li M, Firestone GL, Bjeldanes LF. 2008. 3,3′-Diindolylmethane stimulates murine immune function in vitro and in vivo. *J Nutr Biochem,* 19, 336–44.
10. Pedersen BK, Hoffman-Goetz L. 2000. Exercise and the immune system: regulation, integration, and adaptation. *Physiol Rev,* 80, 1055–81.
11. Barak Y. 2006. The immune system and happiness. *Autoimmun Rev,* 5, 523–7.
12. Cohen S, Alper CM, Doyle WJ, Treanor JJ, Turner RB. 2006. Positive emotional style predicts resistance to illness after experimental exposure to rhinovirus or influenza a virus. *Psychosom Med,* 68, 809–15.
13. Glaser R, Kennedy S, Lafuse WP, et al. 1990. Psychological stress-induced modulation of interleukin 2 receptor gene expression and interleukin 2 production in peripheral blood leukocytes. *Arch Gen Psychiatry,* 47, 707–12.
14. Galbo H. 1983. *Hormonal and Metabolic Adaptation to Exercise.* New York, NY: Thieme Verlag.
15. Volek JE, Kramer WJ, Bush JA, et al. 1997. Testosterone and cortisol in relationship to dietary nutrients and resistance exercise. *J Appl Physiol,* 82, 49–54.
16. Kujala UM, Alen M, Huhtaniemi IT. 1990. Gonadotrophin-releasing hormone and human chorionic gonadotrophin tests reveal that both hypothalamic and testicular endocrine functions are suppressed during acute prolonged physical exercise. *Clin Endocrinol,* 33, 219–25.
17. Ryden M, Hedback B, Jonasson L. 2009. Does stress reduction change the levels of cortisol secretion in patients with coronary artery disease? *J Cardiopulmonary Rehab Prev,* 29, 314–17.

CHAPTERS 20, 21, AND 22: CURRENT CONTROVERSIES AND QUESTIONS

1. Gates TJ. 2001. Screening for cancer: Evaluating the evidence. *Am Fam Physician,* 63, 513–22.
2. Kwabi-Addo B, Ozen M, Ittmann M. 2004. The role of fibroblast growth factors and their receptors in prostate cancer. *Endocr Relat Cancer,* 11, 709–24.
3. Yin M, Bastacky S, Chandran U, Becich MJ, Dhir R. 2008. Prevalence of incidental prostate cancer in the general population: a study of healthy organ donors. *J Urol,* 179, 892–5.
4. Hessels D, Verhaegh GW, Schalken JA, Witjes JA. 2004. Applicability of biomarkers in the early diagnosis of prostate cancer. *Expert Rev Mol Diagn,* 4, 513–26.
5. Austoker J. 1994. Screening for ovarian, prostatic, and testicular cancers. *BMJ,* 309, 315–20.

6. Schroder FH, Hugosson J, Roobol MJ, et al. 2009. Screening and prostate-cancer mortality in a randomized European study. *N Engl J Med,* 360, 1320–8.

7. Walter LC, Bertenthal D, Lindquist K, Konety BR. 2006. PSA screening among elderly men with limited life expectancies. *JAMA,* 296, 2336–42.

8. Green BB, Taplin SH. 2003. Breast cancer screening controversies. *J Am Board Fam Pract,* 16, 233–41.

9. Shen Y, Parmigiani G. 2005. A model-based comparison of breast cancer screening strategies: mammograms and clinical breast examinations. *Cancer Epidemiol Biomarkers Prev,* 14, 529–32.

10. Smith JJ, Berg CD. 2008. Lung cancer screening: promise and pitfalls. *Semin Oncol Nurs,* 24, 9–15.

11. Beane J, Sebastiani P, Whitfield TH, et al. 2008. A prediction model for lung cancer diagnosis that integrates genomic and clinical features. *Cancer Prev Res (Phila Pa),* 1, 56–64.

12. Schiffman M, Castle PE. 2005. The promise of global cervical-cancer prevention. *N Engl J Med,* 353, 2101–4.

13. Wallace MB, Kemp JA, Trnka YM, Donovan JM, Farraye FA. 1998. Is colonoscopy indicated for small adenomas found by screening flexible sigmoidoscopy? *Ann Intern Med,* 129, 273–8.

14. Chan-Smutko G, Patel D, Shannon KM, Ryan PD. 2008. Professional challenges in cancer genetic testing: who is the patient? *Oncologist,* 13, 232–8.

15. Wakefield CE, Meiser B, Homewood J, Ward R, O'Donnell S, Kirk J. 2008. Randomized trial of a decision aid for individuals considering genetic testing for hereditary nonpolyposis colorectal cancer risk. *Cancer,* 113, 956–65.

16. Hartge P, Struewing JP, Wacholder S, Brody LC, Tucker MA. 1999. The prevalence of common BRCA1 and BRCA2 mutations among Ashkenazi Jews. *Am J Hum Genet,* 64, 963–70.

17. Hudson KL. 2007. Prohibiting genetic discrimination. *N Engl J Med,* 356, 2021–3.

18. Michels KB, Giovannucci E, Chan AT, Singhania R, Fuchs CS, Willett WC. 2006. Fruit and vegetable consumption and colorectal adenomas in the Nurses' Health Study. *Cancer Res,* 66, 3942–53.

19. Bjelakovic G, Nikolova D, Gluud LL, Simonetti RG, Gluud C. 2007. Mortality in randomized trials of antioxidant supplements for primary and secondary prevention: systematic review and meta-analysis. *JAMA,* 297, 842–57.

20. Lee SH, Oe T, Blair IA. 2001. Vitamin C-induced decomposition of lipid hydroperoxides to endogenous genotoxins. *Science,* 292, 2083–6.

21. Feiz HR, Mobarhan S. 2002. Does vitamin C intake slow the progression of gastric cancer in Helicobacter pylori-infected populations? *Nutr Rev,* 60, 34–6.

22. Proteggente AR, Rehman A, Halliwell B, Rice-Evans CA. 2000. Potential problems of ascorbate and iron supplementation: pro-oxidant effect in vivo? *Biochem Biophys Res Commun,* 277, 535–40.

23. Wactawski-Wende J, Kotchen JM, Anderson GL, et al. 2006. Calcium plus vitamin D supplementation and the risk of colorectal cancer. *N Engl J Med,* 354, 684–96.

24. Lappe JM, Travers-Gustafson D, Davies KM, Recker RR, Heaney RP. 2007. Vitamin D and calcium supplementation reduces cancer risk: results of a randomized trial. *Am J Clin Nutr,* 85, 1586–91.

25. Ahn J, Peters U, Albanes D, et al. 2008. Serum vitamin D concentration and prostate cancer risk: a nested case-control study. *J Natl Cancer Inst,* 100, 796–804.

26. Davis CD. 2008. Vitamin D and cancer: current dilemmas and future research needs. *Am J Clin Nutr,* 88 (suppl), 565S–9S.

27. Moan J, Porojnicu AC, Dahlback A, Setlow RB. 2008. Addressing the health benefits and risks, involving vitamin D or skin cancer, of increased sun exposure. *Proc Natl Acad Sci, USA,* 105, 668–73.

28. Hercberg S. 2005. The history of beta-carotene and cancers: from observational to intervention studies. What lessons can be drawn for future research on polyphenols? *Am J Clin Nutr,* 81 (suppl), 218S–22S.

29. Messina MJ, Wood CE. 2008. Soy isoflavones, estrogen therapy, and breast cancer risk: analysis and commentary. *Nutr J,* 7, 17.

30. Iwasaki M, Inoue M, Otani T, et al. 2008. Plasma isoflavone level and subsequent risk of breast cancer among Japanese women: a nested case-control study from the Japan Public Health Center–based prospective study group. *J Clin Oncol,* 26, 1677–83.

31. Park Y, Hunter DJ, Spiegelman D, et al. 2005. Dietary fiber intake and risk of colorectal cancer: a pooled analysis of prospective cohort studies. *JAMA,* 294, 2849–57.

32. Lupton JR. 2004. Microbial degradation products influence colon cancer risk: the butyrate controversy. *J Nutr,* 134, 479–82.

33. Chung FL, Schwartz J, Herzog CR, Yang YM. 2003. Tea and cancer prevention: studies in animals and humans. *J Nutr,* 133, 3268S–74S.

34. United States Department of Agriculture, Economic Research Service. 2010. Adoption of genetically engineered crops in the U.S. http://www.ers.usda.gov/Data/Biotech Crops/ (accessed Jan. 3, 2011).

35. Union of Concerned Scientists. 2002. Risks of genetic engineering. http://www.ucsusa. org/food_and_agriculture/science_and_impacts/impacts_genetic_engineering/risks-of-genetic-engineering.html (accessed Jan. 4, 2011).

36. Dona A, Arvanitoyannis IS. 2009. Health risks of genetically modified foods. *Crit Rev Food Sci Nutr,* 49, 2, 164–75.

37. Bakshi A. 2003. Potential adverse health effects of genetically modified crops. *J Toxicol Environ Health B Crit Rev,* 6, 211–25.

38. Lemaux PG. 2008. Genetically engineered plants and foods: a scientist's analysis of the issues (Part I). *Annu Rev Plant Biol,* 59, 771–812.

39. Benedet JL, Anderson GH, Matisic JP. 1992. A comprehensive program for cervical cancer detection and management. *Am J Obstet Gynecol,* 166, 1254–9.

40. Henson DE, Block G, Levine M. 1991. Ascorbic acid: biologic functions and relation to cancer. *J Natl Cancer Inst,* 146, 231–43.

41. Duarte TL, Lunec J. 2005. Review: when is an antioxidant not an antioxidant: a review of novel actions and reactions of vitamin C. *Free Radic Res,* 39, 671–86.

42. Carr A, Frei B. 1999. Does vitamin C act as a pro-oxidant under physiological conditions? *FASEB J,* 13, 1007–24.

43. Zeeb H, Greinert R. 2010. The role of vitamin D in cancer prevention. *Deutsches Arzteblatt International,* 107, 638–43.

44. Affenito SG, Kerstetter J. 1999. Position of the American Dietetic Association and Dietitians of Canada: Women's Health and Nutrition. *J Am Diet Assoc,* 99, 738–51.

45. Duffy C, Perez K, Partridge A. 2007. Implications of phytoestrogen intake for breast cancer. *CA Cancer J Clin,* 57, 260–77.
46. Maliakal PP, Coville PF, Wanwimolruk S. 2001. Tea consumption modulates hepatic drug metabolising enzymes in Wistar rats. *J Pharm Pharmacol,* 53; 4, 569–77.
47. Khan SG, Katiyar SK, Agarwal R, Mukhtar H. 1992. Enhancement of anti-oxidant and phase II enzymes by oral feeding of green tea polyphenols in drinking water to SKH-1 hairless mice: possible role in cancer chemoprevention. *Cancer Res,* 52, 4050–2.
48. Yang CS, Liao J, Yang GY, Lu G. 2005. Inhibition of lung tumorigenesis by tea. *Exp Lung Res,* 31, 135–44.
49. Sadava D, Whitlock E, Kane SE. 2007. The green tea polyphenol, epigallacatechin-3-gallate inhibits telomerase and induces apoptosis in drug-resistant lung cancer cells. *Biochem Biophys Res Commun,* 360, 233–7.
50. Zheng W, Doyle TJ, Kushi LH, Sellers TA, Hong CP, Folsom AR. 1996. Tea consumption and cancer incidence in a prospective cohort study of postmenopausal women. *Am J Epidemiol,* 144, 175–82.
51. Nagano J, Kono S, Preston DL, Mabuchi K. 2001. A prospective study of green tea consumption and cancer incidence. Hiroshima and Nagasaki (Japan). *Cancer Causes Control,* 12, 501–8.
52. Li Q, Kakizaki M, Kuriyama S, et al. 2008. Green tea consumption and lung cancer risk: the Ohsaki study. *Br J Cancer,* 99, 1179–84.
53. Mirick DK, Davis S, Thomas DB. 2002. Antiperspirant use and the risk of breast cancer. *J Natl Cancer Inst,* 94(20), 157–80.
54. Cancer Research UK. 2011. Cancer questions and answers: Deodorants, antiperspirants and breast cancer. http://www.cancerhelp.org.uk/about-cancer/cancer-questions/deodorants-antiperspirants-and-breast-cancer (accessed Dec. 10, 2010).
55. Cancer and the environment: what you need to know; what you can do, August 2003, National Cancer Institute, U.S. Department of Health and Human Services.
56. Alavanja MCR, Dosemeci M, Samanic C, Lubin J, et al. 2004. Pesticides and lung cancer risk in the agricultural health study cohort. *Am J Epidemiol,* 160, 876–85.
57. National Cancer Institute. 2008. Psychological stress and cancer: Questions and answers. http://www.cancer.gov/cancertopics/factsheet/Risk/stress (accessed Jan. 5, 2011).
58. Spilsberg B, Rundberget T, Johannessen L, Kristoffersen A, Holst-Jensen A, Berdal K. 2010. Detection of food-derived damaged nucleosides with possible adverse effects on human health using a global adductomics approach. *J Agric Food Chem,* 58, 6370–5.
59. National Cancer Institute. 2009. Artificial sweeteners and cancer. http://www.cancer.gov/cancertopics/factsheet/Risk/artificial-sweeteners#ref1 (accessed Dec. 9, 2010).
60. The INTERPHONE Study Group. 2010. Brain tumour risk in relation to mobile telephone use: Results of the INTERPHONE international case-control study. *Int J Epidemiol,* published online ahead of print May 17, 2010.
61. Lonn S, Ahlbom A, Hall P, Feychting M. 2004 Mobile phone use and the risk of acoustic neuroma. *Epidemiology,* 15(6), 653–9.
62. Ahlbom A, Day N, Feychting M, et al. 2000. A pooled analysis of magnetic fields and childhood leukaemia. *Br J Cancer,* 83(5), 692–8.

63. Kheifets L, Ahlbom A, Crespi CM, et al. 2010. Pooled analysis of recent studies on magnetic fields and childhood leukemia. *Br J Cancer,* 103, 1128–35.
64. Linet MS, Hatch EE, Kleinerman RA, et al. 1997. Residential exposure to magnetic fields and acute lymphoblastic leukemia in children. *New Engl J Med,* 337(1), 1–7.
65. He K, Zhao L, Daviglus ML, et al. 2008. Association of monosodium glutamate intake with overweight in Chinese adults: the INTERMAP study. *Obesity,* 16, 1875–80.
66. Geha RS, Beiser A, Ren C, Patterson R, et al. 2000. Review of alleged reaction to monosodium glutamate and outcome of a multicenter double-blind placebo-controlled study. *J Nutr,* 130, 1058S–62S.
67. Freeman M. 2006. Reconsidering the effects of monosodium glutamate: a literature review. *J Am Acad Nurse Pract,* 18, 482–6.
68. Jinap S, Hajeb P. 2010 Glutamate: Its applications in food and contribution to health. *Appetite,* 55, 1–10.
69. Peters JC, Lawson KD, Middleton SJ, et al. 1997. Assessment of the nutritional effects of olestra, a nonabsorbed fat replacement: summary. *J Nutr,* 127, 1719S–28S.
70. Prince DM, Welschenbach MA. 1998. Olestra: a new food additive. *J Am Diet Assoc,* 98, 565–9.
71. Neuhouser ML, Rock CL, Kristal AR, et al. 2006. Olestra is associated with slight reductions in serum carotenoids but does not markedly influence serum fat-soluble vitamin concentrations. *Am J Clin Nutr,* 83, 624–31.
72. Levine A. 1997. Food fight in Indianapolis. *U.S. News & World Report,* 5, 53–4.
73. Sandler RS, Zorich NL, Filloon TG, et al. 1999. Gastrointestinal symptoms in 3181 volunteers ingesting snack foods containing olestra or triglycerides. *Ann Intern Med,* 130, 253–61.
74. Centers for Disease Control and Prevention. 2009. Irradiation of food: Frequently asked questions. http://www.cdc.gov/nczved/divisions/dfbmd/diseases/irradiation_food/ (accessed Dec. 17, 2010).
75. Centers for Disease Control and Prevention. 2011. CDC estimates of foodborne illness in the United States. http://www.cdc.gov/foodborneburden/2011-foodborne-estimates.html (accessed Dec. 17, 2010).
76. Farkas J. 1998. Irradiation as a method for decontaminating food: A review. *Int J Food Microbiol,* 44, 189–204.
77. Gosse RF, Hartwig DH, Miesch ME, et al. 2002. Food-borne radiolytic compounds (2-alkylcyclobutanones) may promote experimental colon carcinogenesis. *Nutr Cancer,* 44, 189–191.
78. Sommers CH. 2003. 2-Dodecyclobutanone does not induce mutations in the Escherichia coli tryptophan reverse mutation assay. *J Agric Food Chem,* 51, 6367–70.
79. Wood OB, Bruhn CM. 2000. Position of the American Dietetic Association: Food irradiation. *J Am Diet Assoc,* 100, 246–53.
80. Johansen C, Boice JD, McLaughlin JK, et al. 2001. Cellular telephones and cancer—a nationwide cohort study in Denmark. *JNCI,* 93, 203–7.
81. Schuz J, Jacobson R, Olsen JH, et al. 2006. Cellular telephone use and cancer risk: Update of a nationwide Danish cohort. *JNCI,* 98, 1707–13.

82. Sadetzki S, Chetrit A, Freedman L, et al. 2005. Long-term follow-up for brain tumor development after childhood exposure to ionizing radiation for tinea capitis. *Radiat Res,* 163, 424–32.

83. Kundi M. 2009. The controversy about a possible relationship between mobile phone use and cancer. *Environ Health Perspect,* 117, 316–24.

84. Malagoli C, Fabbi S, Teggi S, et al. 2010. Risk of hematological malignancies associated with magnetic fields exposure from power lines: A case-control study in two municipalities of northern Italy. *Environmental Health,* 9, 16–23.

85. Kroll ME, Swanson J, Vincent TJ, Draper GJ. 2010. Childhood cancer and magnetic fields from high-voltage power lines in England and Wales: A case-control study. *Br J Cancer,* 103, 1122–7.

86. Fews AP, Henshaw DL, Wilding RJ, Keitch PA. 1999. Corona ions from powerlines and increased exposure to pollutant aerosols. *Int. J Radiat Biol,* 75, 1523–31.

87. Holden RJ, Pakula JS, et al. 1998. An immunological model connecting the pathogenesis of stress, depression and carcinoma. *Med Hypotheses,* 51, 309–14.

88. Darbre PD. 2009. Underarm antiperspirants/deodorants and breast cancer. *Breast Cancer Res,* 11, S5.

89. Clapp RW, Howe GK, Jacobs MM. 2005. Environmental and occupational causes of cancer: a review of scientific literature. Lowell Center for Sustainable Production. http://www.healthyenvironmentforkids.ca/sites/healthyenvironmentforkids.ca/files/cpche-resources/Cancer_and_the_Environment.pdf (accessed Apr. 10, 2011).

90. U.S. Preventive Services Task Force Recommendation Statement 2009. Screening for breast cancer. *Ann Intern Med,* 151, 716–26.

91. Roos PH, Jakubowski N. 2010. Methods for the discovery of low-abundance biomarkers for urinary bladder cancer in biological fluids. *Bioanalysis,* 2(2), 295–309.

92. Obermayr E, Sanchez-Cabo F, Tea MK, et al. 2010. Assessment of a six gene panel for the molecular detection of circulating tumor cells in the blood of female cancer patients. *BMC Cancer,* 10, 666.

93. Rosas SL, Koch W, da Costa Carvalho MG, et al. 2001. Promoter hypermethylation patterns of p16, O6-methylguanine-DNA-methyltransferase, and death-associated protein kinase in tumors and saliva of head and neck cancer patients. *Cancer Res,* 61, 939–42.

94. CBC News. 2011. Blood test for cancer a step nearer. The Associated Press. http://www.cbc.ca/canada/british-columbia/story/2011/01/03/health-cancer-blood-test.html#ixzz1A0qxPVhd (accessed January 2011).

95. Nagrath S, Sequist LV, Maheswaran S, et al. 2007. Isolation of rare circulating tumor cells in cancer patients by microchip technology. *Nature,* 450, 1235–9.

96. The American Cancer Society. 2009. Fruits and vegetables: Do you get enough? http://www.cancer.org/Healthy/EatHealthyGetActive/EatHealthy/fruits-and-vegetables-do-you-get-enough (accessed Jan. 4, 2011).

97. Block G. 1991. Vitamin C and cancer prevention: The epidemiologic evidence. *Am J Clin Nutr,* 53, 270S–282S.

98. National Cancer Institute. Selenium and vitamin E cancer prevention trial (SELECT), http://www.cancer.gov/newscenter/qa/2008/selectqa (accessed May 2, 2011).

99. Messina M, Persky V, Setchell KD, Barnes S. 1994. Soy intake and cancer risk: A review of the in vitro and in vivo data. *Nutr Cancer,* 21, 113–31.

100. Phillips GO and Cui SW. 2011. An introduction: Evolution and finalization of the regulatory definition of dietary fiber. *Food Hydrocolloids,* 25, 139–43.
101. Bingham SA, Day NE, Luben R, Ferrari P, Slimani N, Norat T et al. 2003. Dietary fibre in food and protection against colorectal cancer in the European Prospective Investigation into Cancer and Nutrition (EPIC): An observational study. *Lancet,* 361, 1496–501.
102. Peters U, Sinha R, Chatterjee N, Subar AF, Ziegler RG, Kulldorff M., et al. 2003. Dietary fibre and colorectal adenoma in a colorectal cancer early detection programme. *Lancet,* 361, 1491–5.
103. The American Cancer Society. 2011. Aspartame. www.cancer.org/Cancer/Cancer-Causes/OtherCarcinogens/AtHome/aspartame (accessed Apr. 6, 2011).
104. Cancer Research UK. 2006. Cancer news: EU rules out aspartame cancer risk. http://info.cancerresearchuk.org/news/archive/cancernews/2006-05-09-eu-rules-out-aspartame-cancer-risk (accessed Apr. 6, 2011).
105. National Cancer Institute. 2006. Fact sheet: Aspartame and cancer. http://www.cancer.gov/cancertopics/factsheet/Risk/aspartame (accessed Apr. 6, 2011).
106. U.S. Department of Agriculture. 2005. Dietary guidelines for Americans. http://www.health.gov/dietaryguidelines/dga2005/document/html/chapter5.htm (accessed Dec. 1, 2010).
107. Lappe JM, Travers-Gustafson D, Davies KM, Recker RR, and Heaney RP. 2008. Vitamin D and calcium supplementation reduces cancer risk: Results of a randomized trial. *Am J Clin Nutr,* 85, 1586–91.
108. Correa P, Fontham ET, Bravo LE, Ruiz B, Zarama G, Realpe JL, et al. 2000. Chemo-prevention of gastric dysplasia: Randomized trial of antioxidant supplements and anti-helicobacter pylori therapy. *J. Natl Cancer Inst,* 92, 1881–88.
109. National Institutes of Health, Office of Dietary Supplements. 2011. Dietary supplement fact sheet: Vitamin D. http://ods.od.nih.gov/factsheets/VitaminD (accessed Jan. 7, 2011).
110. International Agency for Research on Cancer. 2001. Press Release: IARC finds limited evidence that residential magnetic fields increase the risk of childhood leukemia. http://www.iarc.fr/en/media-centre/pr/2001/pr136.html (accessed Mar. 16, 2011).
111. Cancer Research UK. 2009. Dietary factors and breast cancer. http://www.cancerhelp.org.uk/type/breast-cancer/about/diet/dietary-factors-and-breast-cancer#pesticides (accessed Jan. 3, 2011).
112. Cancer Research UK. 2010. Pesticides and cancer. http://info.cancerresearchuk.org/healthyliving/cancercontroversies/pesticides/(accessed Jan. 3, 2011).
113. National Cancer Institute.2010. Lung cancer. www.cancer.gov/cancertopics/types/lung (accessed Apr. 7, 2011).
114. American Cancer Society. 2011. Colorectal cancer overview: How many people get colorectal cancer? http://www.cancer.org/Cancer/ColonandRectumCancer/OverviewGuide/colorectal-cancer-overview-key-statistics (accessed Apr. 7, 2011).
115. World Cancer Research Fund/American Institute for Cancer Research. 1997. Food research and the prevention of cancer: A global perspective. www.aicr.org/site/News2?page=NewsArticle&id=13067 (accessed May 2, 2011).

CONCLUSION

1. Xu J, Kibel AS, Hu JJ, et al. 2009. Prostate cancer risk associated loci in African Americans. *Cancer Epidemiol Biomarkers Prev,* 18, 2145–9.
2. Ambs S, Marincola FM, Thurin M. 2008. Profiling of immune response to guide cancer diagnosis, prognosis, and prediction of therapy. *Cancer Res,* 68, 4031–3.
3. Yeatman TJ, Mule J, Dalton WS, Sullivan D. 2008. On the eve of personalized medicine in oncology. *Cancer Res,* 68, 7250–2.
4. Weinstein IB, Case K. 2008. The history of cancer research: introducing an AACR centennial series. *Cancer Res,* 68, 6861–2.
5. GLOBOCAN 2008. 2010. Cancer incidence and mortality worldwide, estimated cancer deaths for 2010. http://globocan.iarc.fr/burden.asp?selection_pop=220900&Text-p=World&selection_cancer=280&Text-c=All+cancers+excl.+non-melanoma+skin+cancer&pYear=2&type=1&window=1&submit=%A0Execute%A0 (accessed Apr. 6, 2011).
6. World Health Organization. 2011. Cancer fact sheet number 297. http://www.who.int/mediacentre/factsheets/fs297/en/ (accessed Apr. 6, 2011).
7. National Institutes of Health (U.S.). 2007. Biological sciences curriculum study: Cancer and society. Bethesda (MD) Bookshelf ID: NBK20362. http://www.ncbi.nlm.nih.gov/books/NBK20362/ (accessed Mar. 18, 2011).
8. National Cancer Institute. 2008. Annual report to the nation finds declines in cancer incidence and death rates. http://www.cancer.gov/newscenter/pressreleases/2008/reportnation2008release (accessed Apr. 14, 2011).
9. National Cancer Institute. Cancer Genome Anatomy Project. http://www.ncbi.nlm.nih.gov/ncicgap/ (accessed Apr. 7, 2011).
10. National Cancer Institute. 2010. TAILORx Breast Cancer Trial http://www.cancer.gov/clinicaltrials/noteworthy-trials/tailorx (accessed Apr. 7, 2011).
11. Moffitt Cancer Center. 2011. Overview: What is total cancer care? http://www.moffitt.org/totalcancercare (accessed Apr. 7, 2011).
12. UN News Center. 2010. New cancer cases and deaths to double by 2030. http://www.un.org/apps/news/story.asp?NewsID=34888&Cr=world+health+organization&Cr1 (accessed Apr. 7, 2011).

Index

radiation exposure, 57; tobacco smoking, 57–58

National Lung Screening Trial (NLST), 160
Neck cancer. *See* Head and neck cancer
Neuroendocrine carcinoma, 103–4. *See also* Skin cancer
Neurofibromatosis (Types 1 and 2), 11. *See also* Brain cancer
Nevoid basal cell carcinoma syndrome, 102–3
NF1/NF2 tumor suppressor gene, 11, 12. *See also* Brain cancer
Nicotine: additives to, 78–79; effects on brain/addiction, 77–78, 81; and smoking, 76–77
NLST (National Lung Screening Trial), 160
Nondiscrimination law, 166
Non-Hodgkin Lymphoma, 60–61
Nonsteroidal anti-inflammatory drugs (NSAIDs), 35
Nutrition, and cancer risk reduction: cruciferous vegetables, 121–22; garlic, 121; green tea, 122–23; selenium, 124–25; soy, 123; tomatoes/tomato phytochemicals, 119–21; vitamin D, 123–24; vitamin E, 125. *See also* Dietary factors; Perceived risk factors

Obesity: body mass index (BMI), 128, 132; body weight maintenance, 129; and breast cancer, 132; calorie restriction, 138–39; and chronic inflammation, 137–38; and colorectal cancer, 133; and diabetes, 87; energy balance, 128; fat consumption, 118; fat location, 131–32; as global epidemic, 127; and pancreatic cancer, 92–93; and physical exercise, 134; socioeconomic link, 131
Occupational exposure: and bladder cancer, 4–5; and brain cancer, 16; and esophageal cancer, 42; and pancreatic cancer, 92
Occupation-associated cancer: environmental carcinogens, 111–12; morbidity/mortality, 109; workplace carcinogens, 109–11

Olestra, 187
Omega-3 polyunsaturated fatty acids, 117
Opium use, 41–42
Oral infection. *See* Periodontitis
Oral sex, 51
Outdoor air pollutants, 111–12
Ovarian cancer: morbidity/mortality, 83; symptoms, 83–84
Ovarian cancer, risk factors: age, 84; diet, 84–85; endometriosis, 87; genetic/hereditary risk factors, 86; growth factors, 85–86; hormonal factors, 85; ionizing radiation exposure, 86–87; Lynch syndrome, 86
Oxidative stress reduction, 136

PAHs (polycyclic aromatic hydrocarbons): and bladder cancer, 5; and esophageal cancer, 40, 42; and head and neck cancer, 53; and tobacco, 79
Pancreatic cancer: and exercise, 135; morbidity/mortality, 89–90; symptoms, 90
Pancreatic cancer, risk factors: age, 90; diet, 93; familial predisposition, 91–92; genetic/hereditary risk factors, 91; obesity/diabetes, 92–93; occupational exposure, 92; tobacco smoke, 90–91
Pancreatitis, 91
Papanicolaou, George, 161
Pap smear screening, 25, 26–27, 161–62
Parasites/parasitic infection, 5
Perceived risk factors: environmental exposure, 188–91; food additives, 185–88; genetically modified organisms (GMOs), 183–85
Periodontitis, 54
Personalized medicine, 198–99
Pesticides. *See* Chemical exposure
P53 tumor suppressor gene: and brain cancer, 11–12; and cervical cancer, 26; and head and neck cancer, 52, 54; and liver cancer, 69; and lung cancer, 79; and prostate cancer, 97; and skin cancer, 197
Phase I drug-metabolizing enzymes, 116
Physical activity/exercise: biological mechanisms for, 135–36; and breast

About the Authors

BERNARD KWABI-ADDO is assistant professor of cancer research and a principal investigator at Howard University in Washington, D.C. Dr. Kwabi-Addo has written many scientific publications in top peer-review journals. He has received several scientific awards, including the American Association for Cancer Research Minority-Serving Institution Faculty Scholar Award. He lives in Virginia.

TIA LAURA LINDSTROM is a freelance writer with an interest in health issues and has coauthored Praeger's *An Introduction to the Work of a Medical Examiner* (2010). She is a graduate of the University of British Columbia and lives in Canada.